Yoga Sutras of Patañjali

ii. Sādhana pāda: chapter on practice

a coloring book by rebecca polack, ph.d.

blū lotus
PUBLICATIONS

First Edition: October 2021

Cover Color Design by Tricia Counce

Paperback: ISBN: 978-1-7373264-1-0

Names: Polack, Rebecca, author.
Subjects: Yoga and Yoga Philosophy. | Indian Philosophy. | Yoga Sūtras of Patañjali.

Printed in the United States of America.
Blū Lotus Publications
www.blulotusbooks.com

To request permission or to purchase in bulk for promotional, educational, or business use, contact the author at rebecca@blulotusbooks.com.

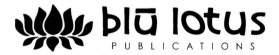

to my mother

❧ introduction ☙

I am a lazy yoga practitioner. Some days I just don't want to practice. There are so many other things that I would rather do. It's avoidance, I admit. But when I step onto my mat, there is no resistance. I start to breathe and slowly begin to move my limbs into a standing forward bend or downward dog, and then I just stay there, sometimes for minutes. I let my body absorb breath and posture. Little movements grow into bigger movements. Slowly more postures begin to form and flow. Slowly my breath increases in length. Slowly my mind becomes uncluttered and calm. There is a sense of ease and joy as my body tunes into the practice. I have often told my students of my laziness, encouraging them to cultivate their own home practice: "If I can practice, the lazy yoga practitioner that I am, then you can practice." One or two postures a day, I tell them. A sun salutation or three. Five minutes sitting with the breath. Just do it, I say.

When I first started practicing so many years ago, I would take one Iyengar Yoga class every week or two. The teacher would guide us through only a few poses, but by the end of the class, I felt buoyant. I would go home and, with gusto, practice everything we did in class for the rest of that week. Every day. It was so liberating to move my body with the precision of the Iyengar method. At first, I couldn't feel the actions in my own body that the teacher was talking about—lifting the inner knee; rotating the thigh; hugging muscles to bone. But as I practiced, I started to experience profound shifts in my mind-body understanding. No part of the body was outside the ken of awareness. I could feel muscles and organs, skin and sinew. I could feel the mind relaxing and detect its agitation. I could feel the breath in relationship to my emotions.

Patañjali says in the first chapter of the *Yoga Sūtras* that practice becomes firmly grounded when continued for a long time without interruption and with devotion (I.14). In the second chapter, *Sādhana Pāda*, the Chapter on Practice, Patañjali proposes a method of practice (*kriyā yoga*) right from the get-go, and it sounds something like a Nike ad: act, reflect, surrender (II.1). It's radical in its simplicity. Without action, nothing happens. Without reflection, action is not clearly understood. Without surrender to the infinite, that understanding doesn't absorb into the depths of the mind and body. Surrender is the key to any transformational practice. In fact, this idea of surrender (*īśvara praṇidhāna*) is so important for Patañjali—master of brevity that he is—he mentions it three times in the *Sādhana Pāda*.

Patañjali further promises the reader that this three-fold process of *kriyā yoga* reduces afflictions and leads to *samādhi*, which from the Sanskrit roots means "to come together," indicating a sense of wholeness or integration. (II.2) *Kriyā yoga* is so uncomplicated, so deceptively simple, yet it packs a punch—reducing suffering and promoting well-being.

The second chapter also contains the widely-known method of practice called *aṣṭāṅga yoga*, or the eight-fold path of yoga. This practice is the blueprint for a total spiritual lifestyle. It includes guidelines on how to interact with the outside world at the social level, *yama*; and how to act with one's internal world, *niyama*. These two, *yama* and *niyama*, function as the ethical and moral foundation from which to proceed on one's spiritual journey. Next, the body, breath and senses are regulated through the practices of *āsana*, *prāṇāyāma*, and *pratyāhāra*. That is, postures, breathing techniques, and control of the sense. Although the final three steps along the eightfold path—that of *dhāraṇā* or concentration, *dhyāna* or meditation, and *samādhi* or integration—are mentioned in the second chapter, Patañjali considers these three in depth in the third chapter of the *Yoga Sūtras*.

Much like Patañjali's *kriyā yoga*, the act of coloring the *Yoga Sūtras* is itself a transformational practice: you color; you reflect as you color; and with a release of expectations, there is transformation. You gain insight, a calm mind, and a peaceful heart. The act of "purposeful" coloring creates the space to go deeper into this profound and enduring text. Color itself activates attention and enhances memory performance, while the simple art of coloring engages the mind, body, and senses. Coloring has been shown to reduce stress and anxiety, improve motor skills and vision, and strengthen focus. It also stimulates different parts of the brain, and cultivates fresh ways of knowing and learning. And just like Patañjali's *kriyā yoga*, the act of coloring encourages the contemplative mode of acting, reflecting, and absorbing.

And finally, this coloring book is chockablock full of real and imagined animals of India and Northern California. I loved creating this book, but discovered in the process that I cannot draw monkeys! I tried in vain, but am so happy with the rest of the creatures that fill these pages, that I am sure the colorist will forgive this omission! Similar to the first book, there are many snakes that grace its contents. This is in deference to Śrī Patañjali, who himself is said to be the incarnation of Adiśeṣa, the immortal snake that formed the divan of the Indian deity, Vishnu.

With affection, I bow to Śrī Patañjali, the great sage and compiler of the *Yoga Sūtras*. I bow also to you, dear fellow colorist. Let this be the continuation of a beautiful journey.

Namaste.

yogena cittasya padena vācāṃ
malaṃ śarīrasya ca vaidyakena
yo'pākarottaṃ pravaraṃ munīnāṃ
patañjaliṃ prāñjalirāṇato'smi ||

With hands pressed reverently together,
I bow to Patañjali, the best of sages,
Who dispels impurities of the mind
With yoga, of speech with grammar,
Of body with medicine.

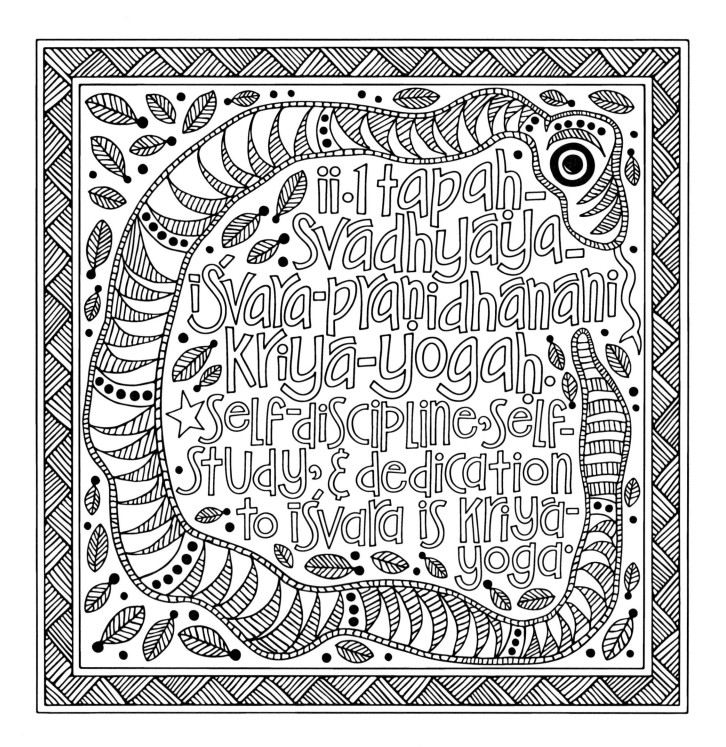

ii.1 tapah-svādhyāya-īśvara-praṇidhānāni kriya-yogah. ☆ self-discipline, self-study, & dedication to īśvara is kriya-yoga.

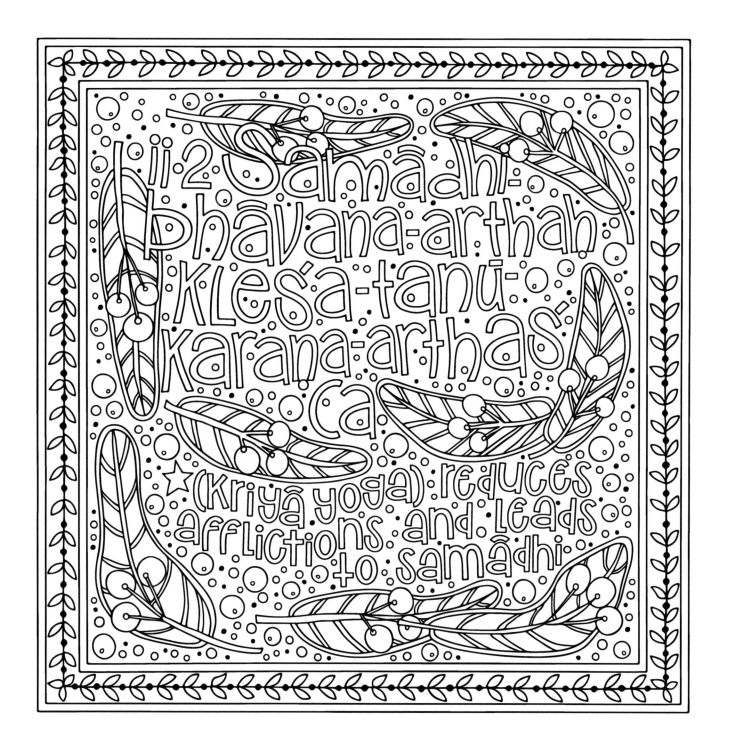

ii.2 Samādhi-bhāvana-arthah klesa-tanū-karana-arthas ca

(Kriyā yoga) reduces afflictions and leads to samādhi

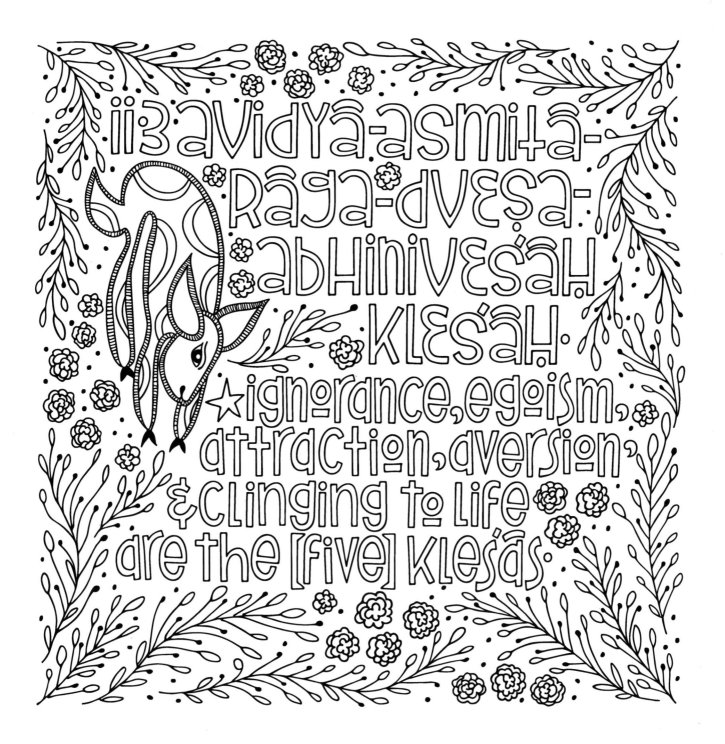

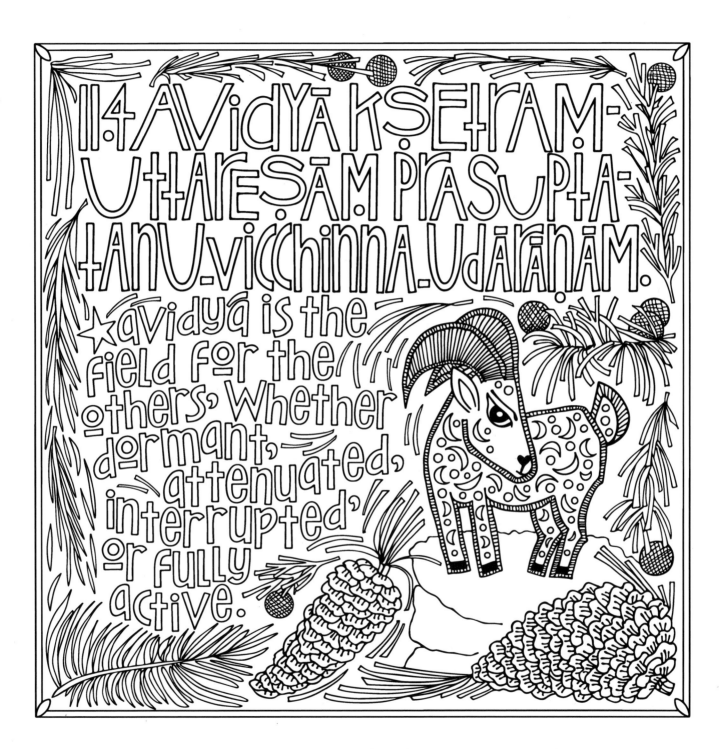

II.4 AVIDYĀ KṢETRAM·
UTTAREṢĀM PRASUPTA·
TANU·VICCHINNA·UDĀRĀNĀM.

★ avidyā is the field for the others, whether dormant, attenuated, interrupted, or fully active.

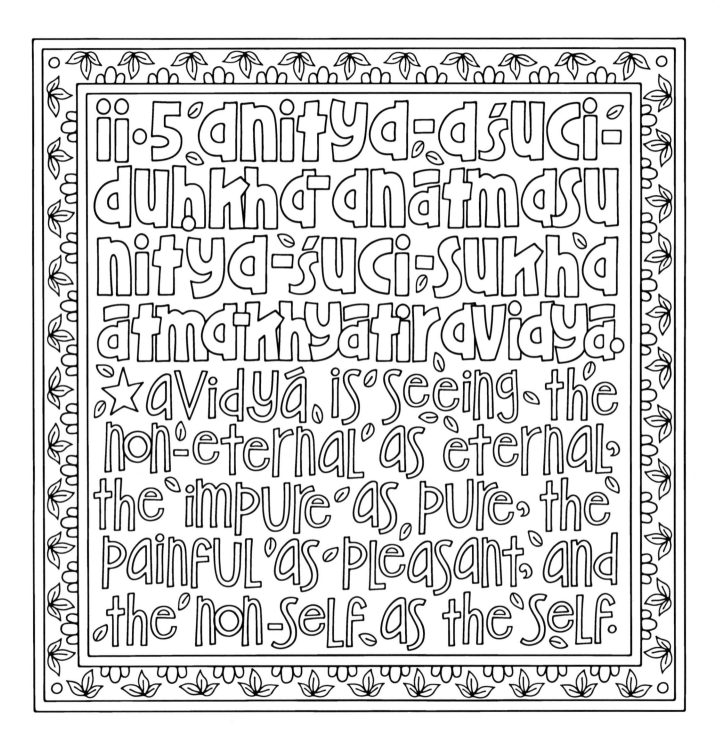

ii.5. anitya-aśuci-duḥkha-anātmasu nitya-śuci-sukha-ātmakhyātiravidyā.

☆ avidyā is seeing the non-eternal as eternal, the impure as pure, the painful as pleasant, and the non-self as the self.

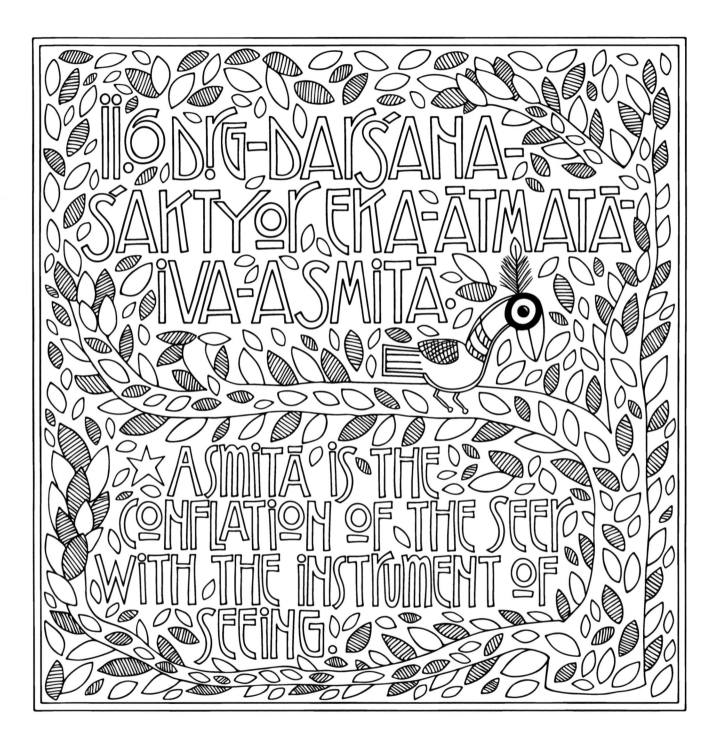

II.6. DṚG-DARŚANA-ŚAKTYOR·EKA-ĀTMATĀ·IVA·ASMITĀ.

ASMITĀ·IS·THE CONFLATION·OF·THE·SEER WITH·THE·INSTRUMENT·OF SEEING.

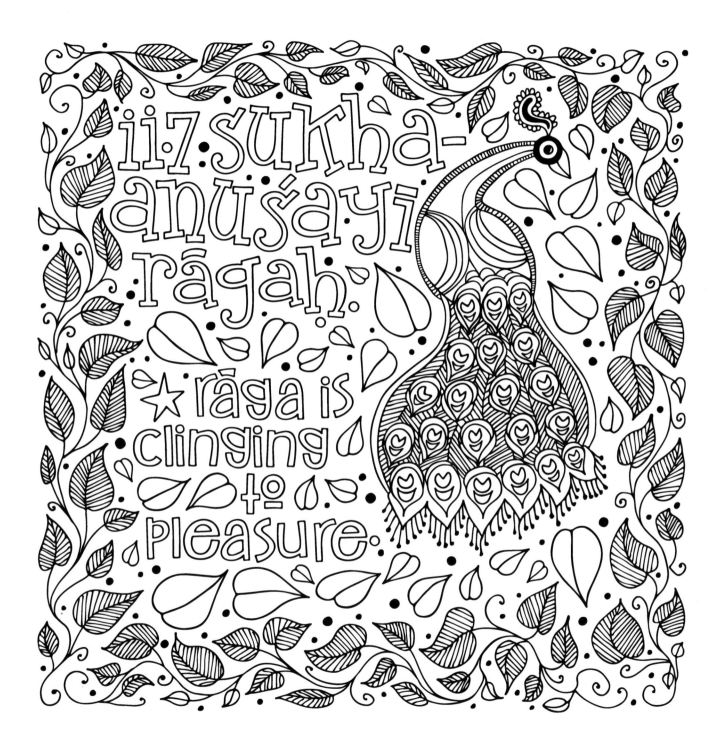

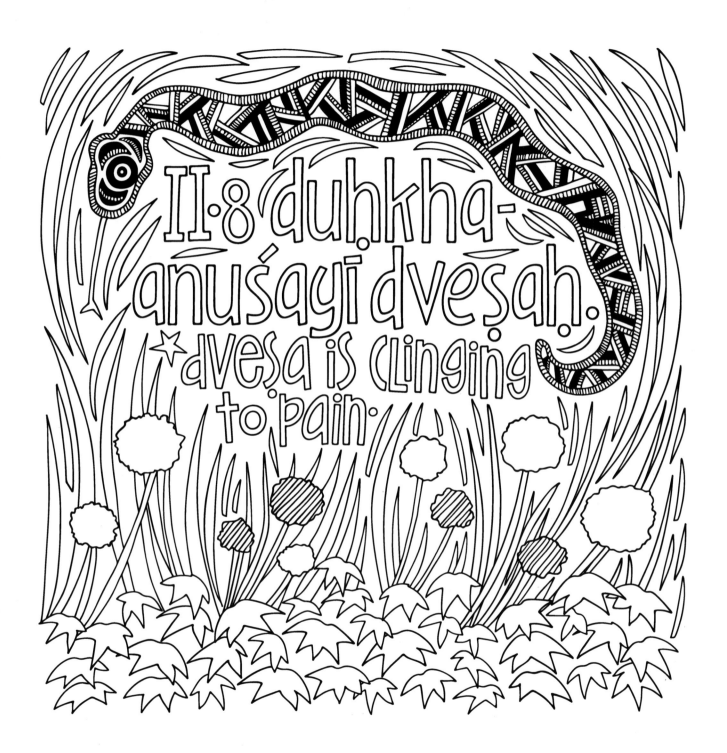

II·8 duḥkha-anuśayi dveṣaḥ. dveṣa is clinging to pain·

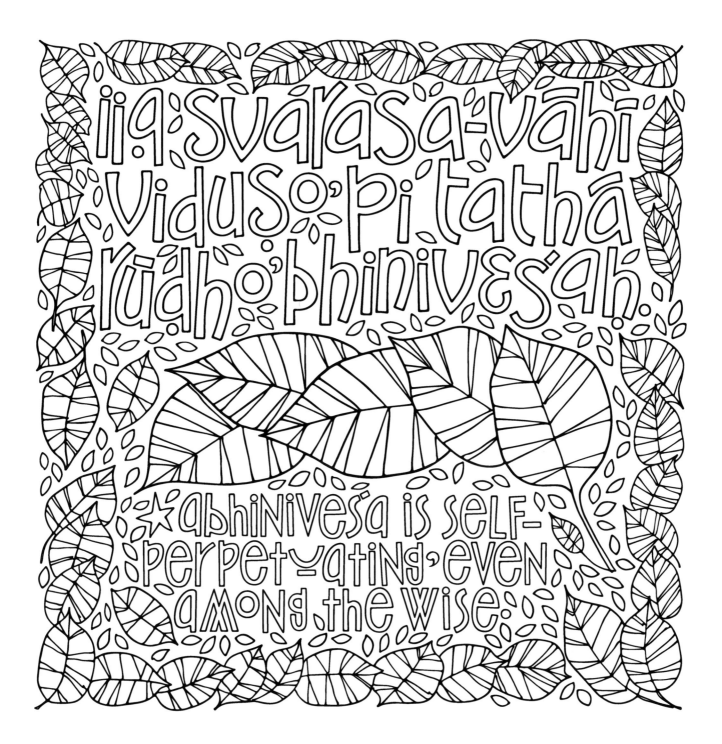

ii.9: svarasā-vāhī
viduṣo'pi tathā
rūḍho'bhiniveśaḥ

abhiniveśa is self-
perpetuating, even
among the wise.

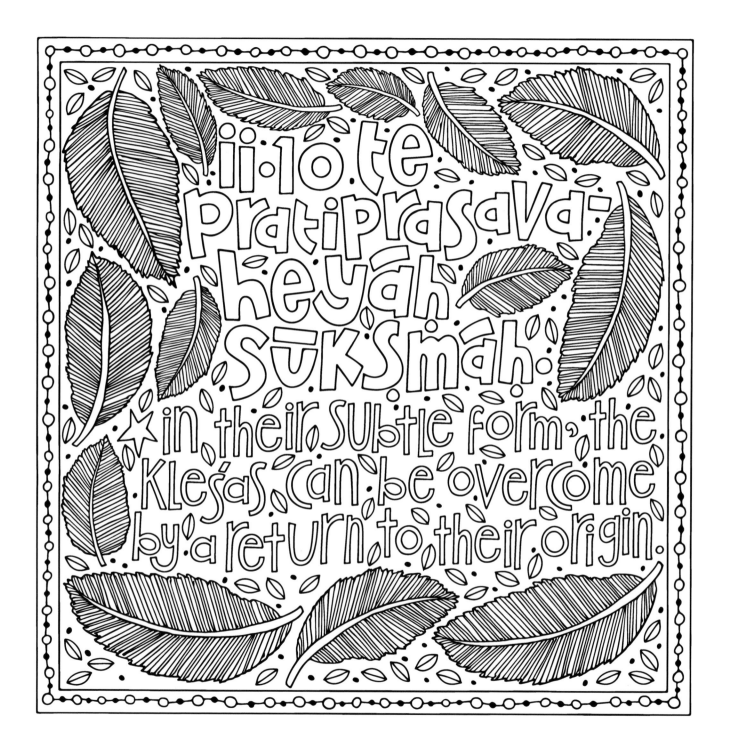

ii·10 te pratiprasava-heyāḥ sūkṣmāḥ.

in their subtle form, the kleśas can be overcome by a return to their origin.

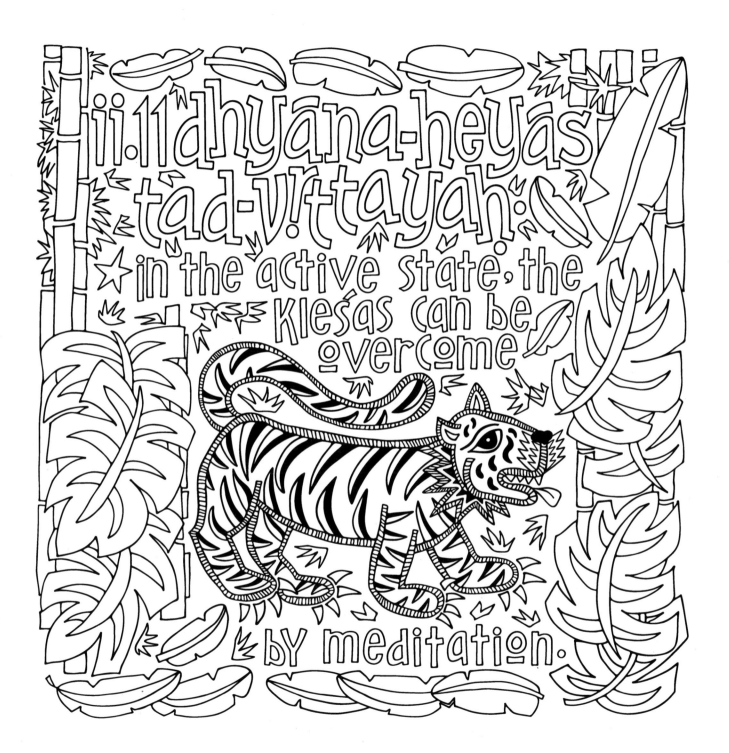

ii.11 dhyāna-heyās tad-vṛttayaḥ:

in the active state, the kleśas can be overcome by meditation.

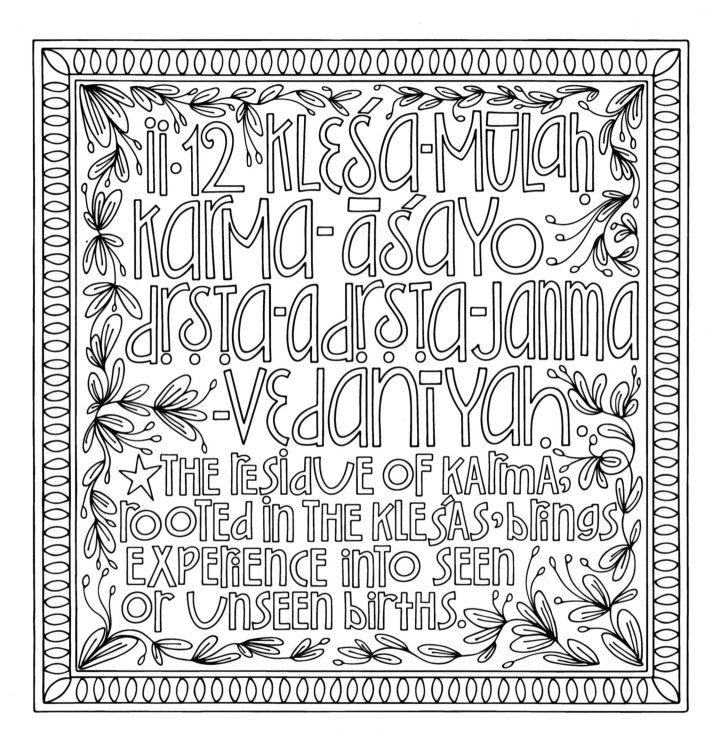

ii.12 kleśa-mūlaḥ
karma-āśayo
dṛṣṭa-adṛṣṭa-janma
-vedanīyaḥ.

★ The residue of karma,
rooted in the kleśas, brings
experience into seen
or unseen births.

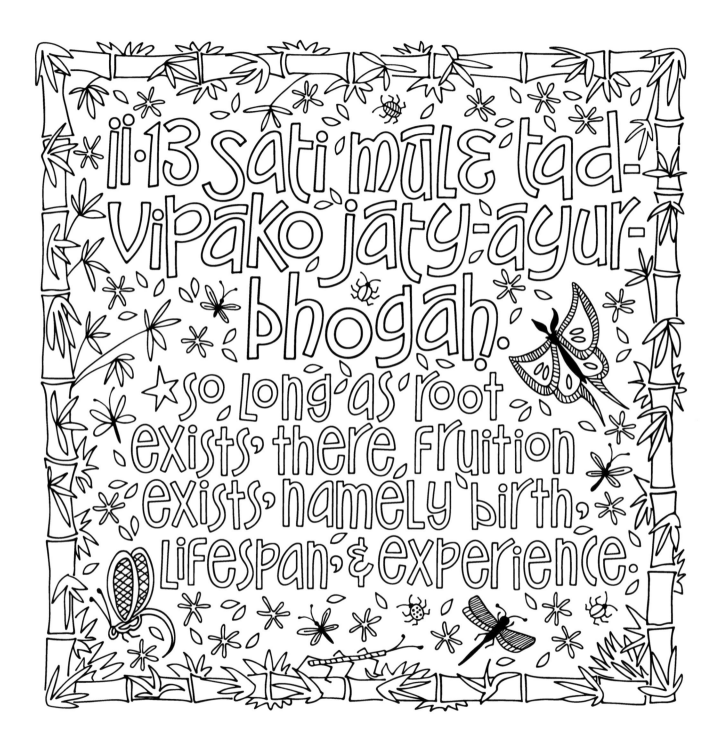

ii·13 sati mūle tad-vipāko jāty-āyur-bhogāḥ.

So long as root exists, there fruition exists, namely birth, lifespan, & experience.

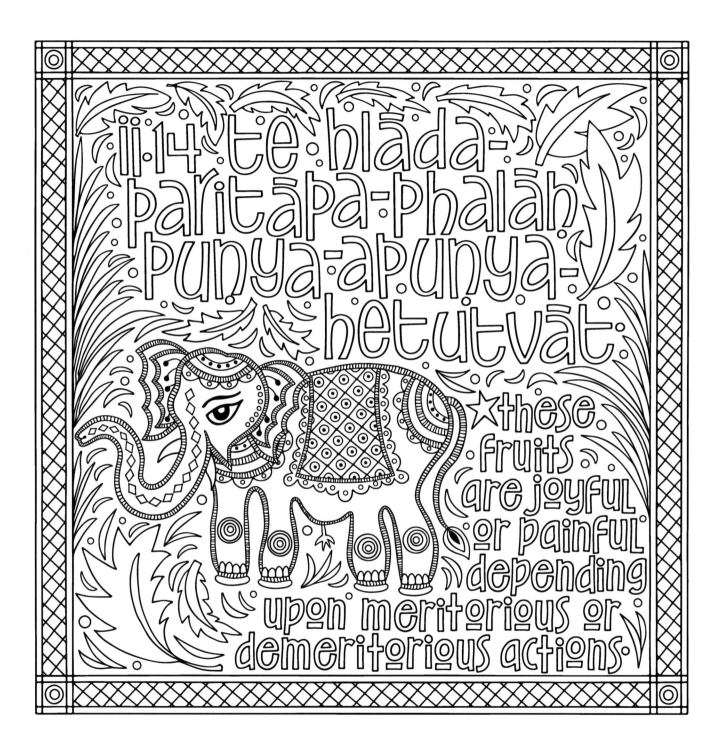

ii·14 te hlāda-
paritāpa-phalāḥ
puṇya-apuṇya-
hetutvāt·

☆these
fruits
are joyful
or painful
depending
upon meritorious or
demeritorious actions·

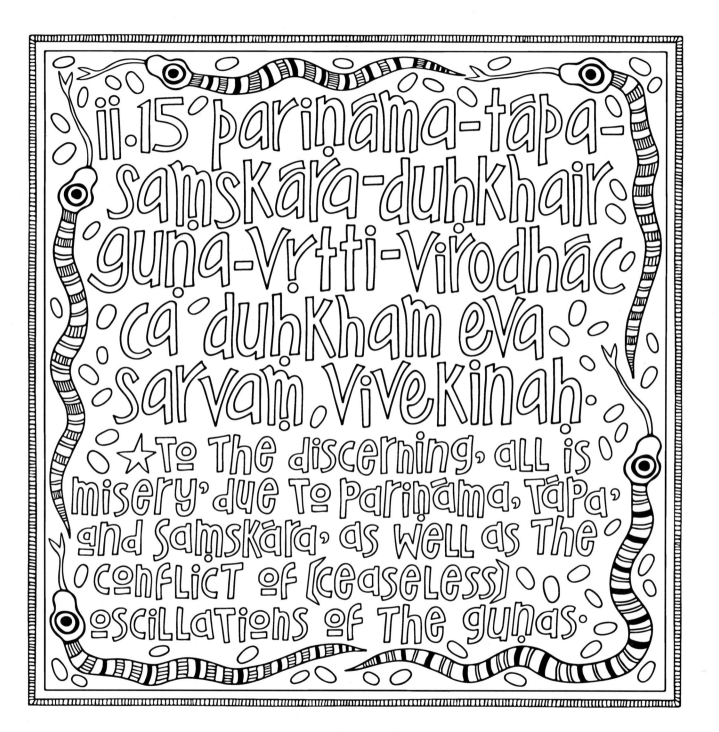

ii.15 pariṇāma-tāpa-saṃskāra-duḥkhair guṇa-vṛtti-virodhāc ca duḥkham eva sarvaṃ vivekinaḥ.

☆ To the discerning, all is misery, due to pariṇāma, tāpa, and saṃskāra, as well as the conflict of (ceaseless) oscillations of the guṇas.

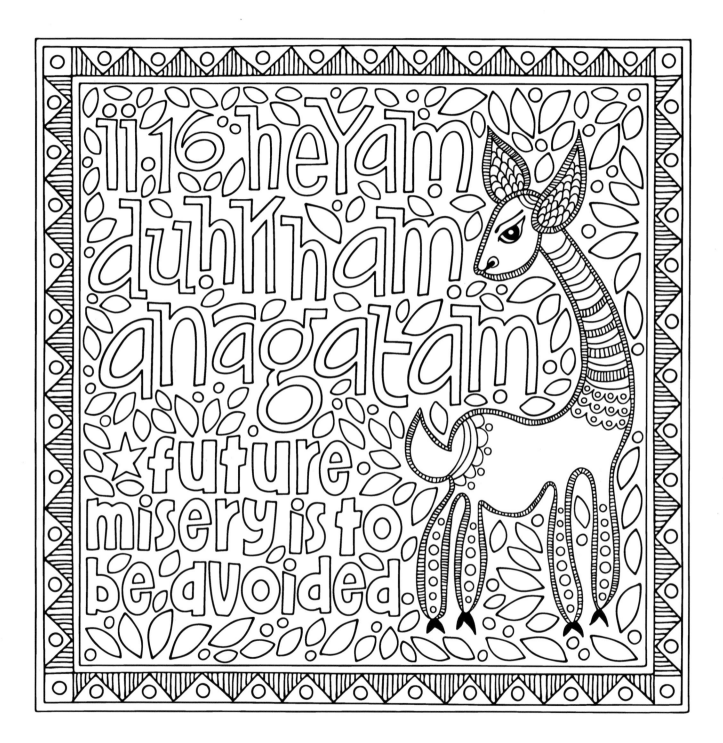

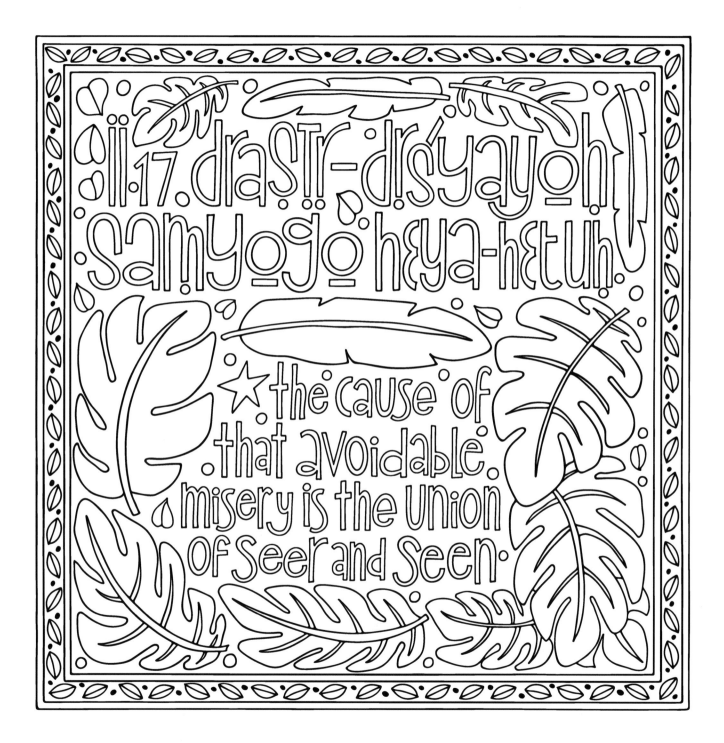

ii.17. draṣṭr-dṛṣ́yayoḥ
saṁyogo heya-hetuḥ.

★ the cause of
that avoidable
misery is the union
of Seer and Seen.

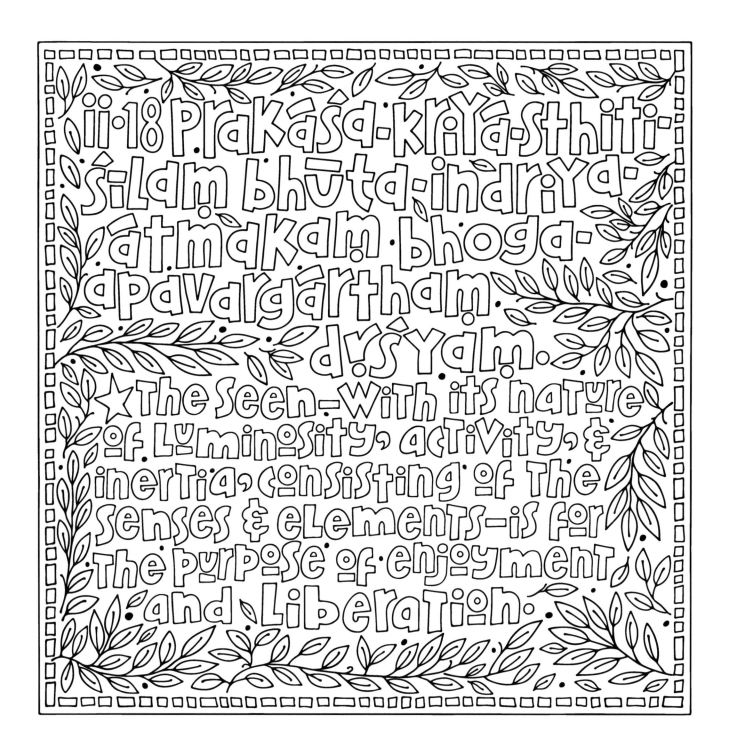

ii.18 prakāśa-kriyā-sthiti-śilam bhūta-indriya-ātmakam bhoga-apavargārtham dṛśyam.

★ The Seen—with its nature of luminosity, activity, & inertia, consisting of the senses & elements—is for the purpose of enjoyment and liberation.

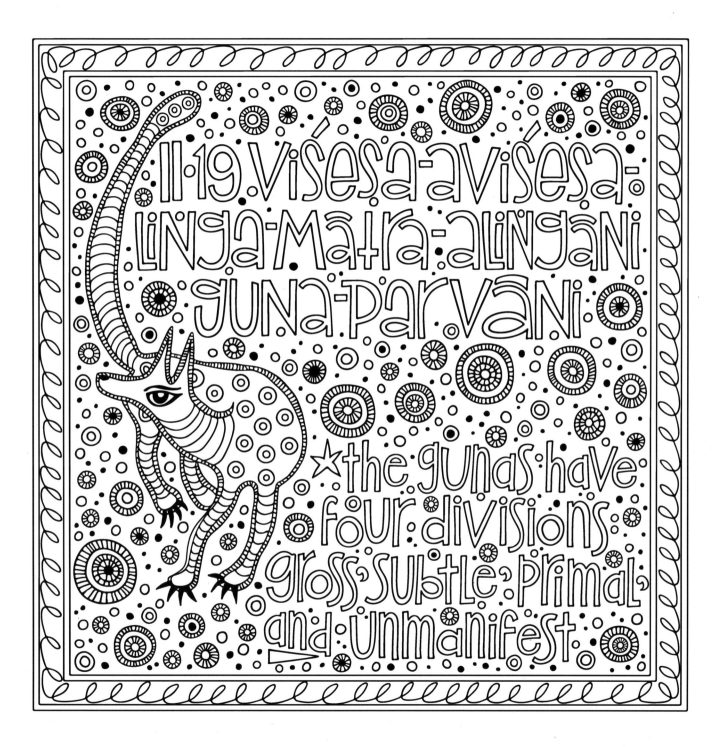

II.19. viśeṣa-aviśeṣa-liṅga-mātra-aliṅgāni guṇa-parvāṇi

★ the guṇas have four divisions: gross, subtle, primal, and unmanifest.

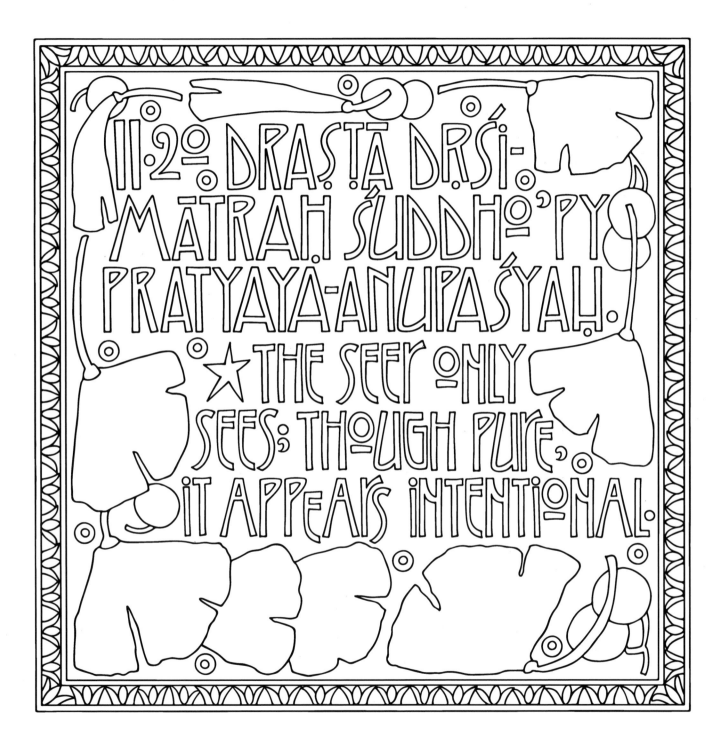

II.20. DRAṢṬĀ DṚŚI-MĀTRAḤ ŚUDDHO 'PY PRATYAYĀ-ANUPAŚYAḤ. ★ THE SEER ONLY SEES; THOUGH PURE, IT APPEARS INTENTIONAL.

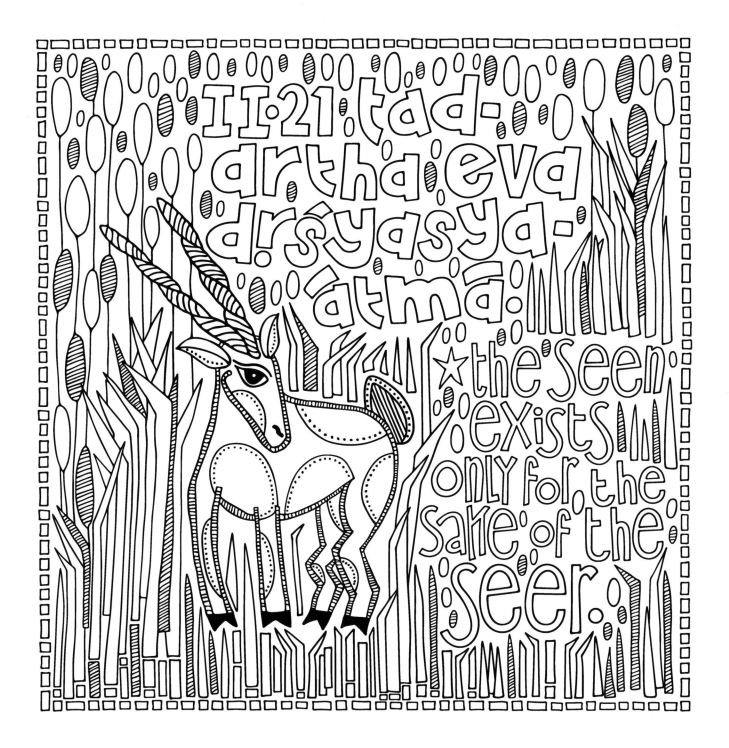

II.21. tad-artha eva dṛśyasyā-ātmā.

the seen exists only for the sake of the seer.

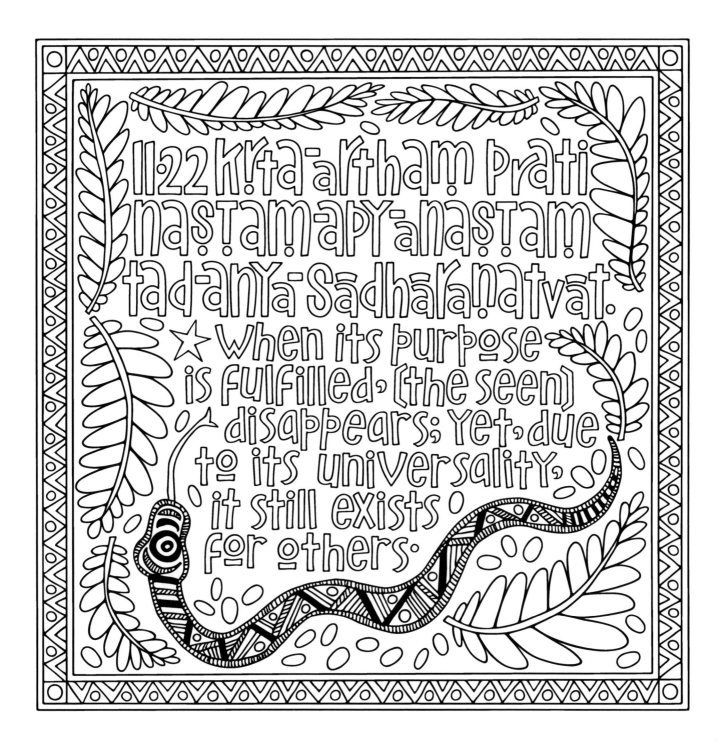

II.22 kṛta-artham prati naṣṭam apy-anaṣṭam tad-anya-sādhāraṇatvāt. ★ When its purpose is fulfilled, (the seen) disappears; yet, due to its universality, it still exists for others.

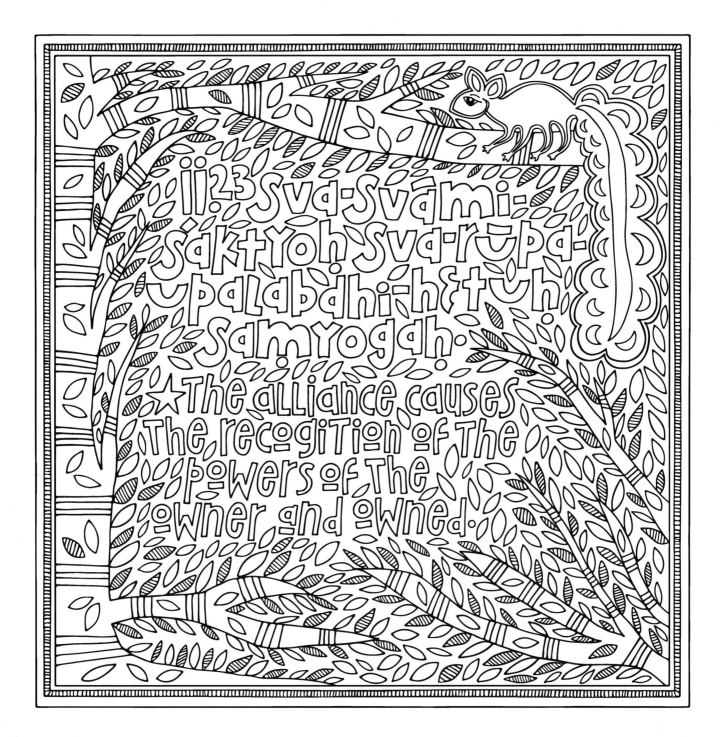

II.23 Sva-Svámi-Śaktyoh Sva-rūpa-Upalabdhi-hetuh Samyogah.

★ The alliance causes the recognition of the powers of the owner and owned.

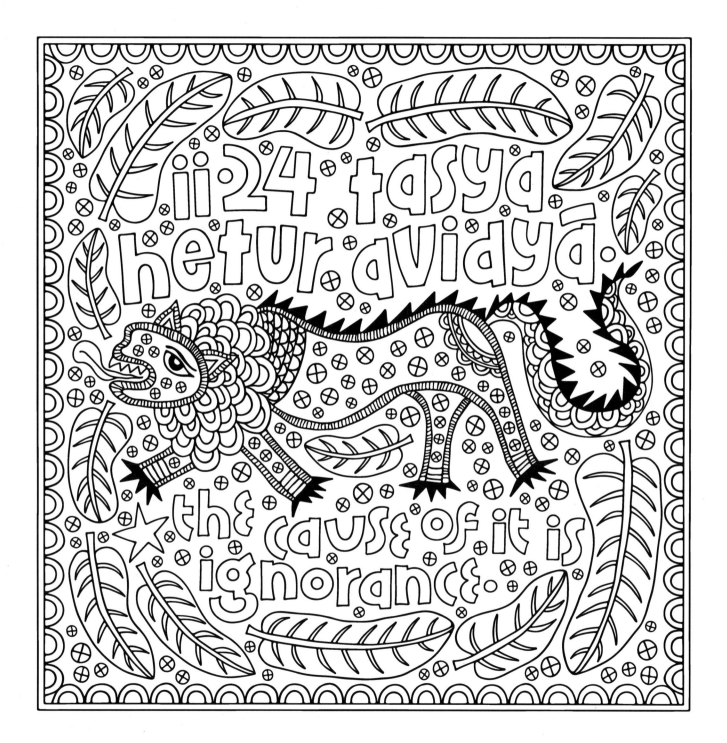

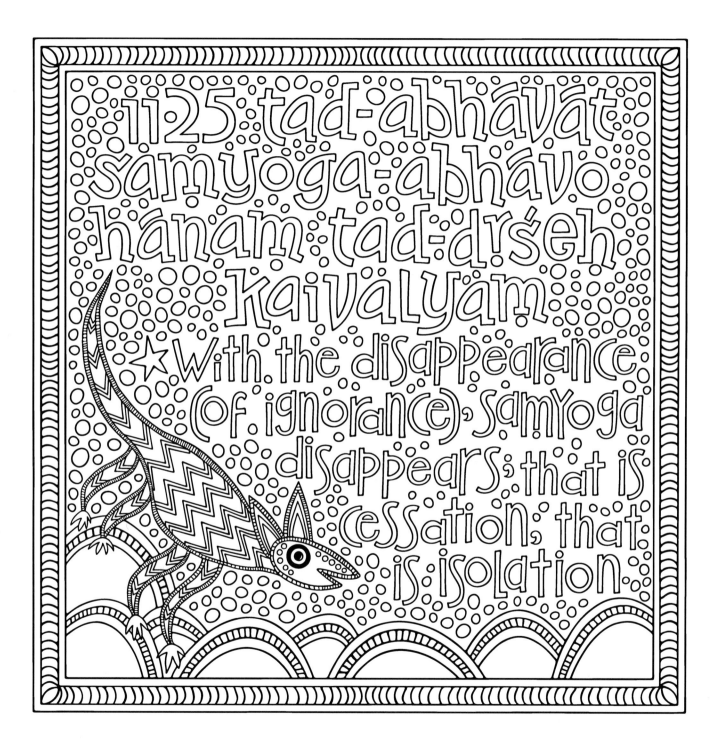

ii25 tad-abhāvāt
saṃyoga-abhāvo
hānam tad-dṛśeh
Kaivālyam
With the disappearance
(of ignorance), saṃyoga
disappears; that is
cessation; that
is isolation.

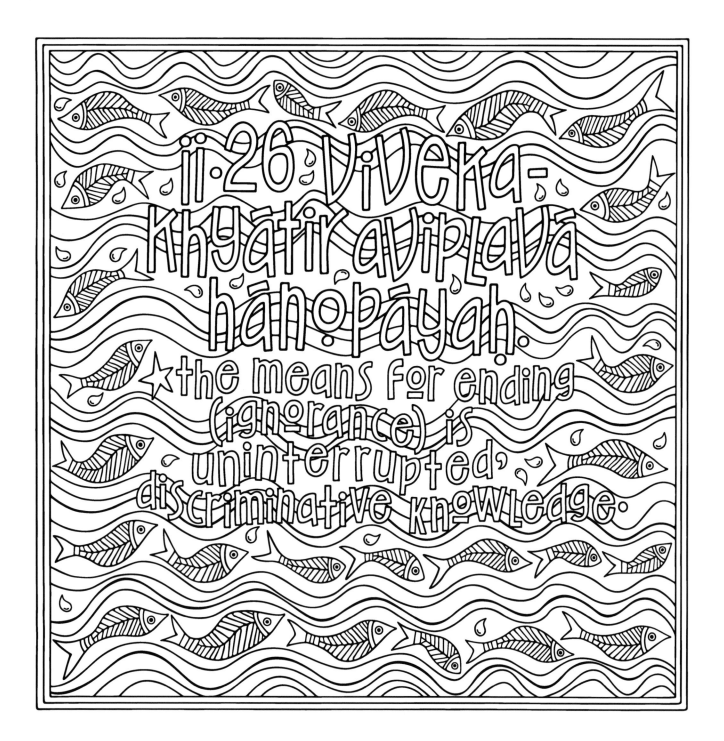

ii.26 viveka-khyatir aviplava hanopayah. ☆ the means for ending (ignorance) is uninterrupted, discriminative knowledge.

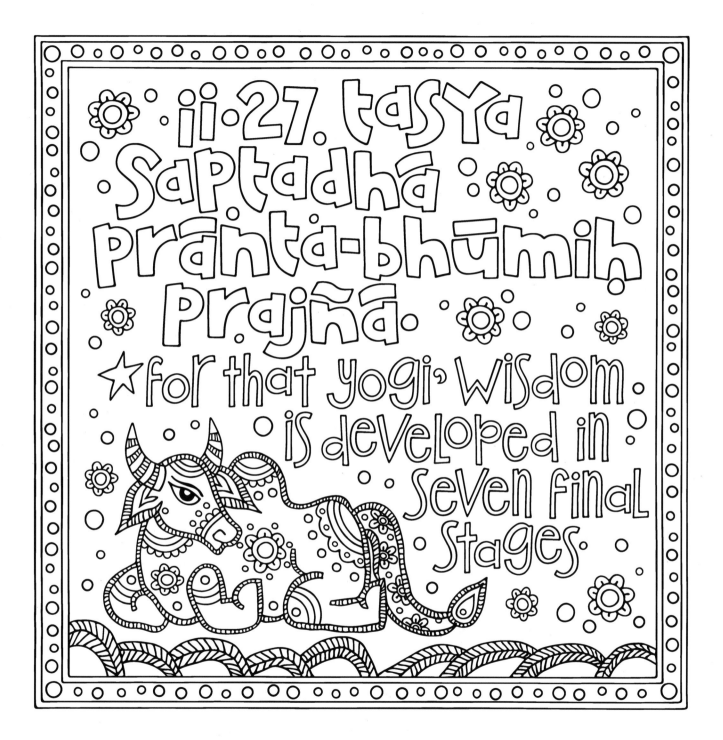

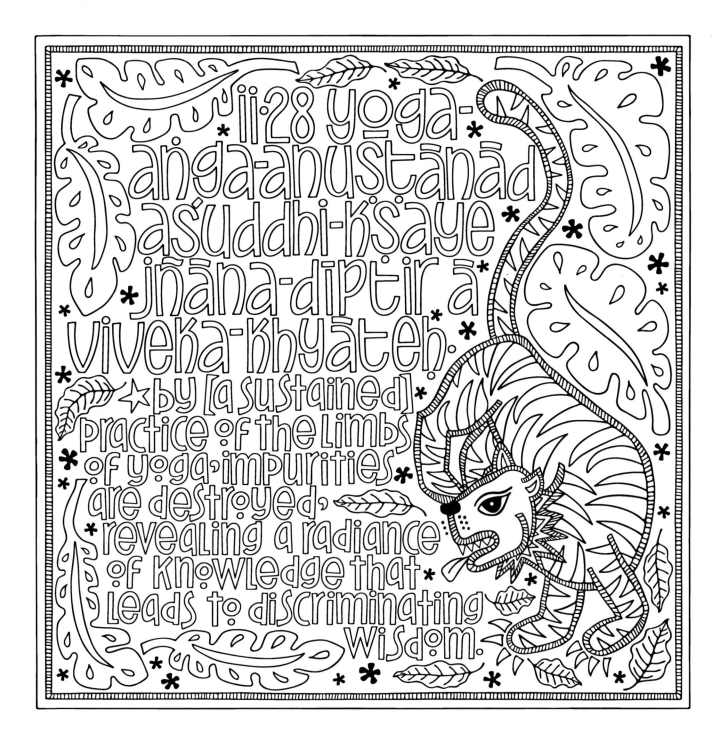

ii.28 yoga-aṅga-anuṣṭānād aśuddhi-kṣaye jñāna-dīptir ā viveka-khyāteḥ.

☆ by [a sustained] practice of the limbs of yoga·impurities are destroyed, revealing a radiance of knowledge that leads to discriminating wisdom.

ii·29 yama-niyama-
asana-pranayama-
pratyahara-dharana-
dhyana-samadhayo
'stav-angani·
☆ restraint, observances,
postures, breath control, sense
withdrawal, concentration,
meditation, & integration
are the eight limbs

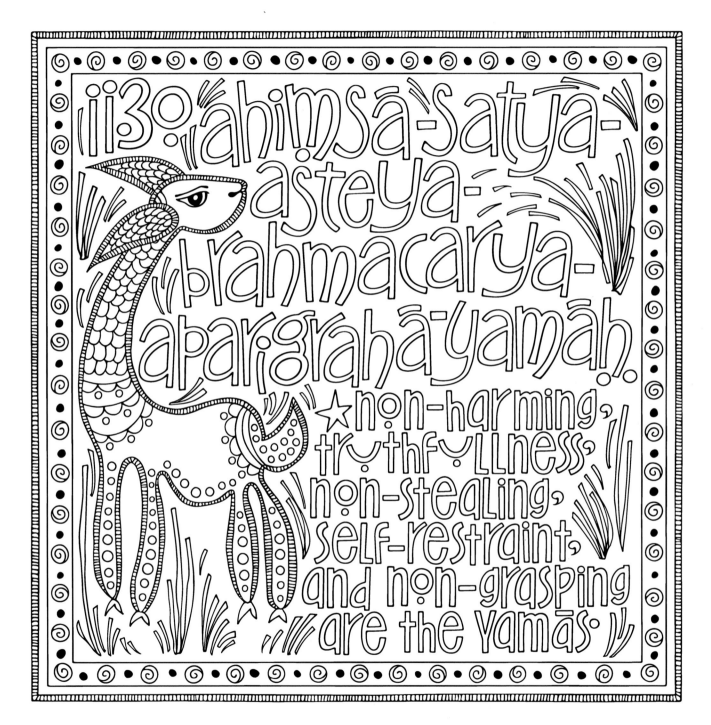

ii30. ahiṃsā-satya-asteya-brahmacarya-aparigrahā yamāḥ.

★non-harming, truthfullness, non-stealing, self-restraint, and non-grasping are the yamās.

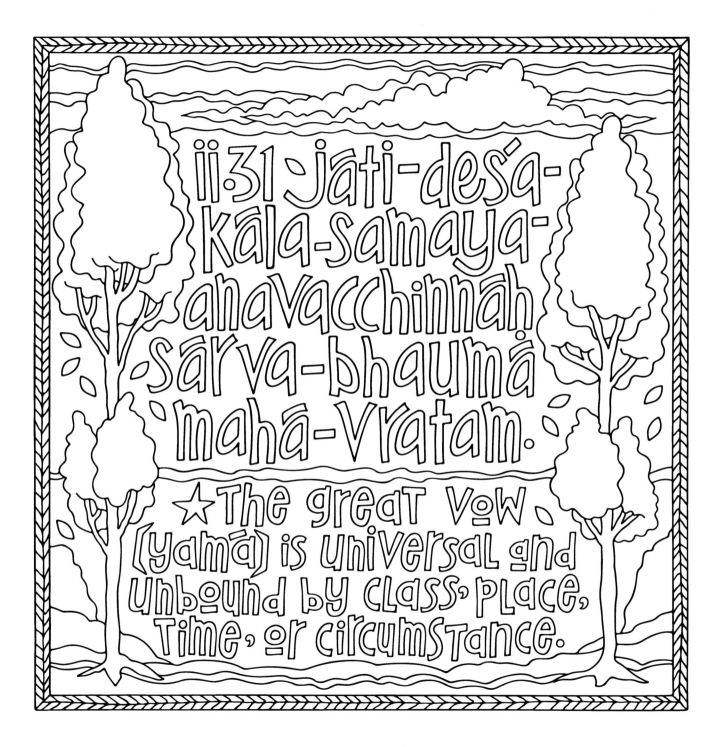

ii·31 jāti-deśa-kāla-samaya-anavacchinnāḥ sārva-bhaumā mahā-vratam.

★ The great vow (yama) is universal and unbound by class, place, time, or circumstance.

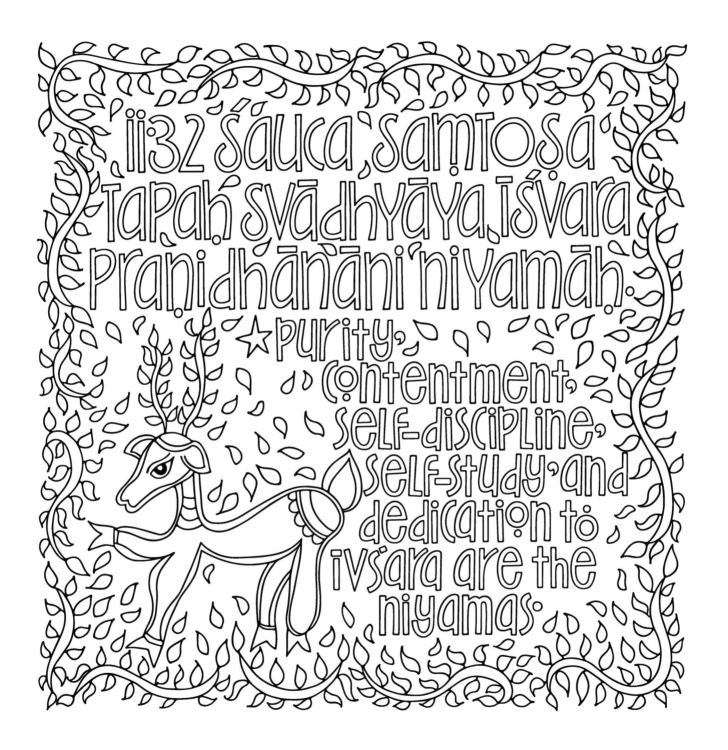

ii32 Śauca, Saṃtoṣa, Tapaḥ Svādhyāya, Īśvara Praṇidhānāni niyamāḥ.

★ purity, contentment, self-discipline, self-study, and dedication to ivsara are the niyamas.

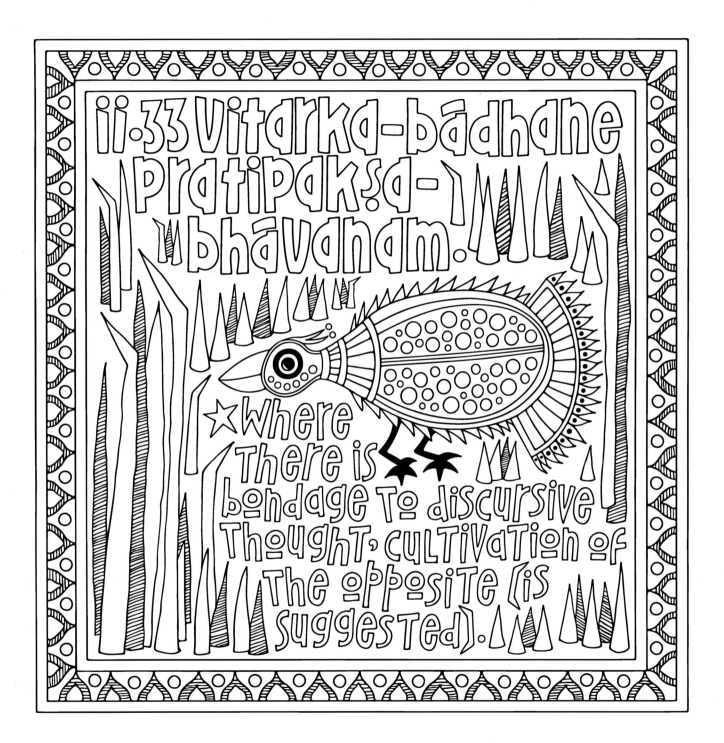

ii·33 vitarka-badhane pratipaksa-bhavanam.

*where there is bondage to discursive thought, cultivation of the opposite (is suggested).

ii.34 vitarkā hiṃsā-ādayaḥ kṛta-kārita-anumoditā lobha-krodha-moha-pūrvakā mṛdu-madhya-adhimātra duḥkha-ajñāna-ananta-phalā iti pratipakṣa-bhāvanam.

☆ negative thoughts—such as violence & the like—whether performed' caused (to be performed)' or authorized' are triggered by greed' anger & delusion; they may be mild' medium' or extreme; they are rooted in ignorance and the source of infinite misery. cultivation of opposite (thoughts is advised).

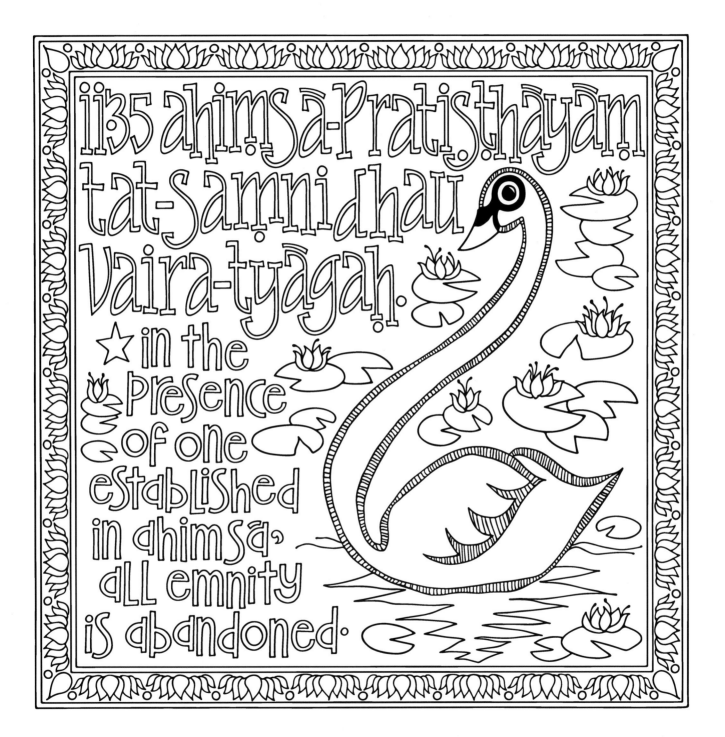

ii35 ahimsā-pratiṣṭhāyāṃ tat-samnidhau vaira-tyāgaḥ.

★ in the presence of one established in ahimsā, all emnity is abandoned.

ii·36·satya·
pratisthayam
kriya·phala·
ashrayatvam·

when established
in satya, there is a
correspondence
between action
and fruit.

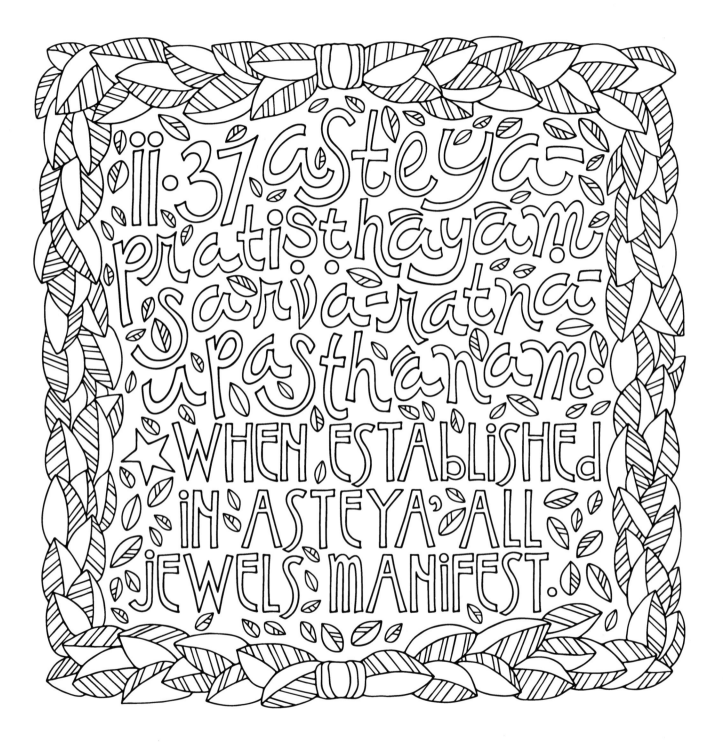

ii.37 asteya-
pratisthayam
sarva-ratna
upasthanam.
WHEN ESTABLISHED
IN 'ASTEYA' ALL
JEWELS MANIFEST.

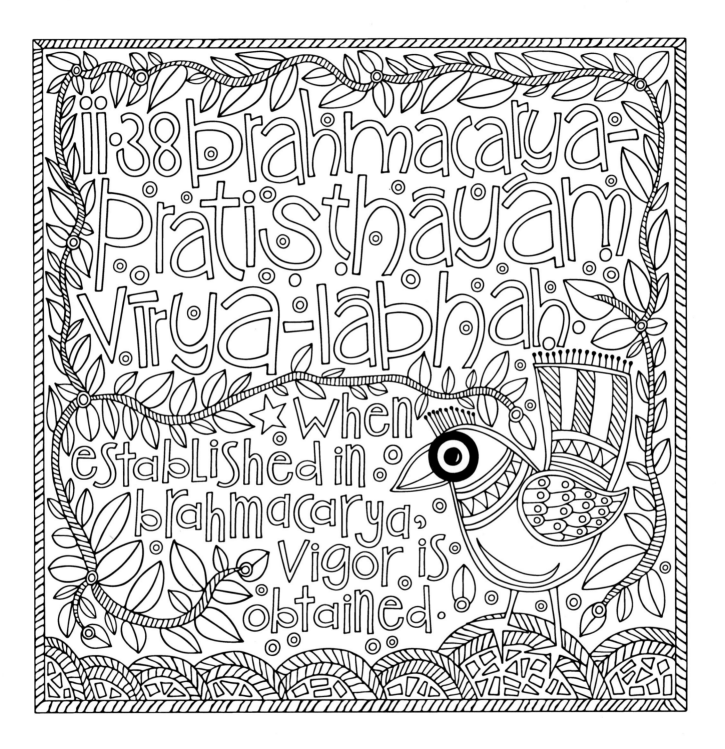

ii.38 brahmacarya-pratiṣṭhāyāṁ vīrya-lābhaḥ.

When established in brahmacarya, vigor is obtained.

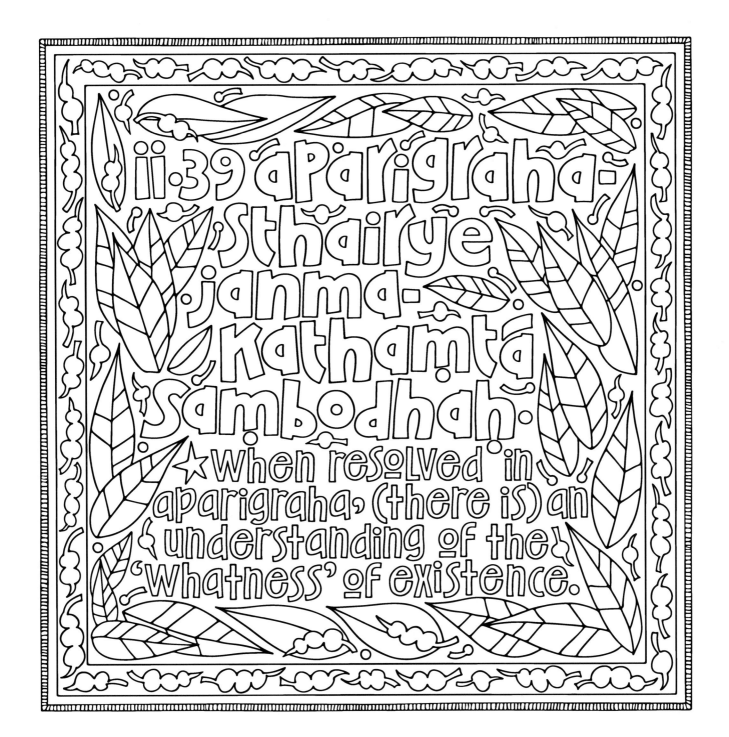

ii.39 aparigraha-
sthairye
janma-
kathamta
sambodhah.
★ when resolved in
aparigraha, (there is) an
understanding of the
'whatness' of existence.

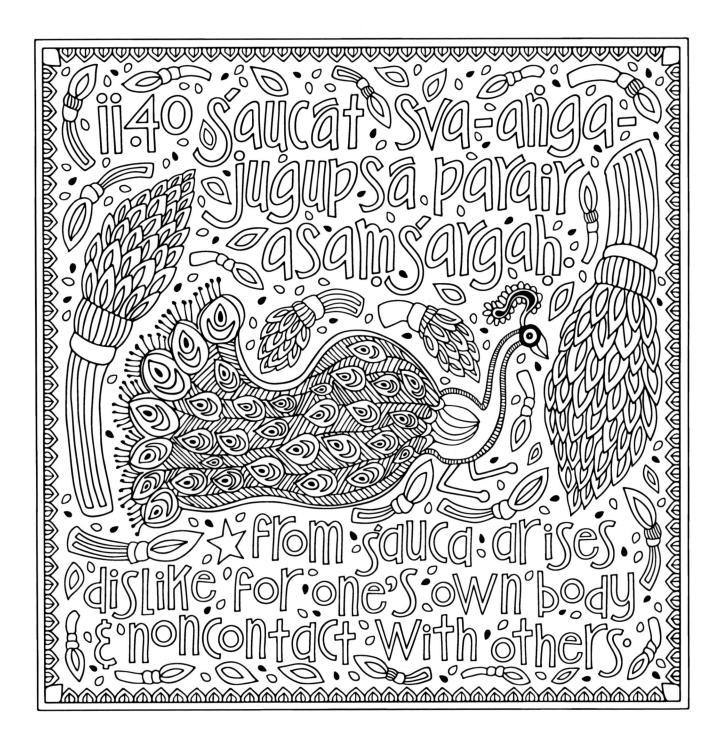

ii.40 śaucāt sva-aṅga-jugupsā parair asaṁsargaḥ

from śauca arises dislike for one's own body & noncontact with others

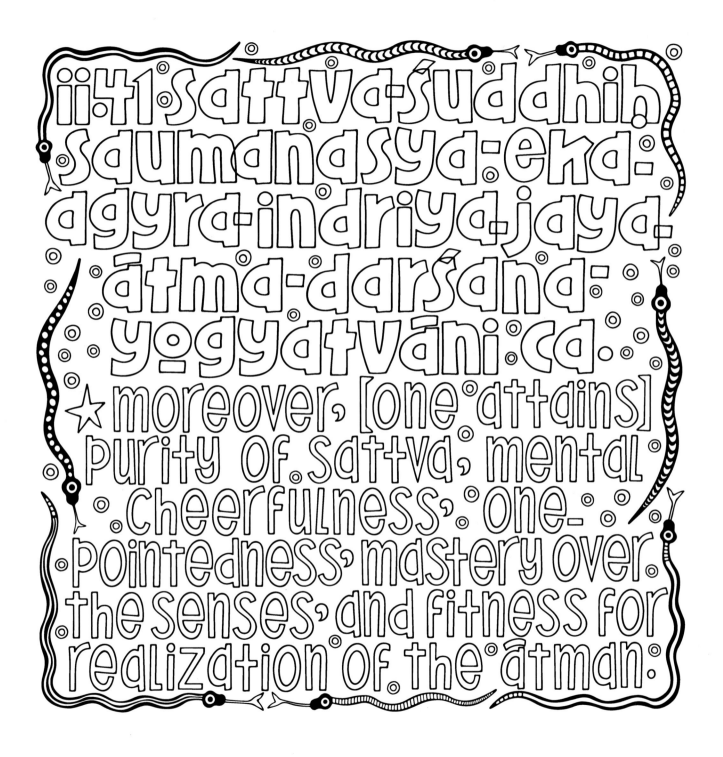

ii.41 sattva-śuddhih saumanasya-eka-agyra-indriya-jaya-ātma-darśana-yogyatvāni ca.

☆ moreover, [one attains] purity of sattva, mental cheerfulness, one-pointedness, mastery over the senses, and fitness for realization of the ātman.

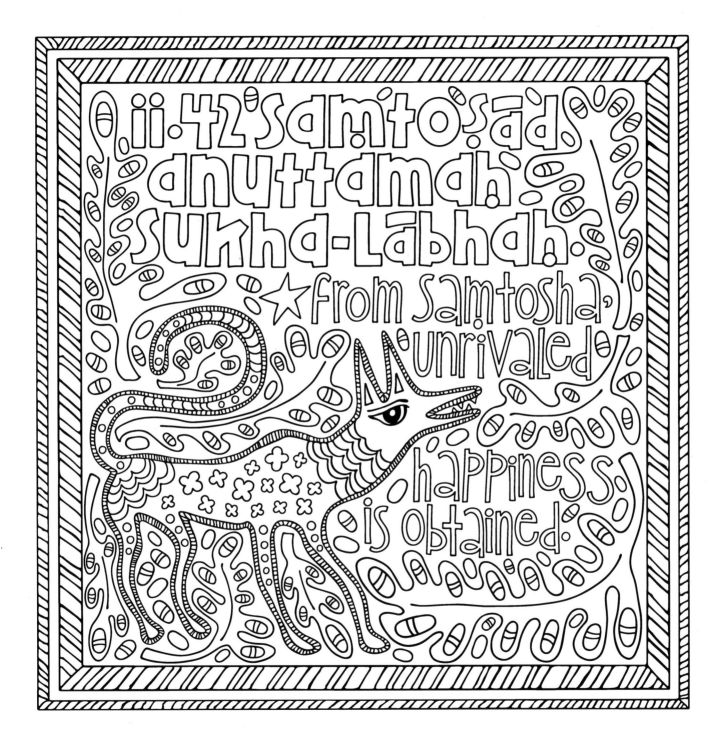

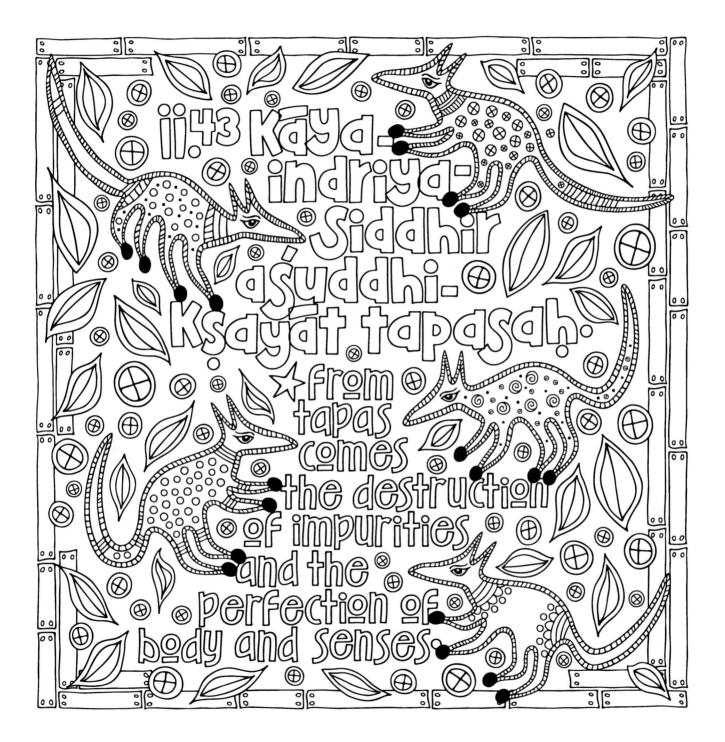

ii.43 Kaya-
indriya-
Siddhir
aśuddhi-
kṣayāt tapasaḥ.

from tapas comes the destruction of impurities and the perfection of body and senses.

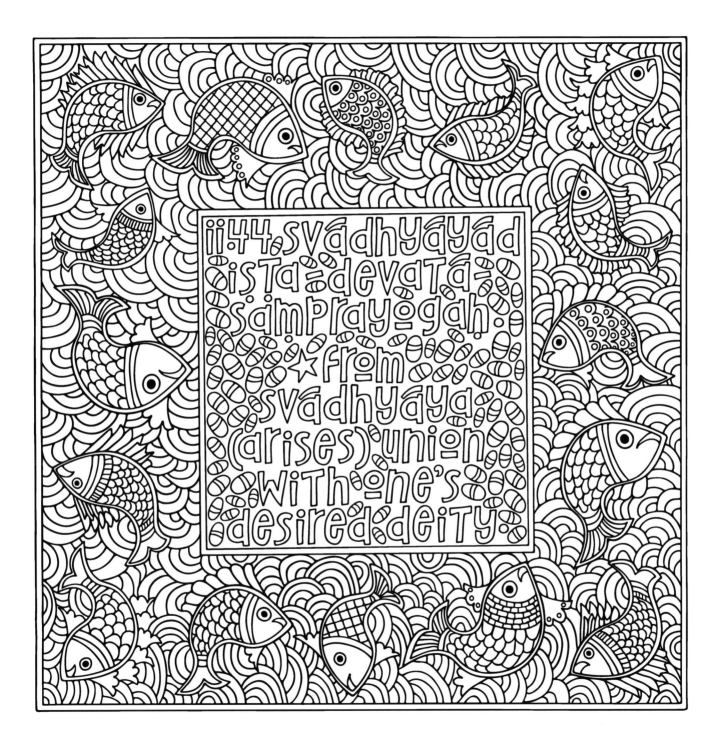

ii.44. svādhyāyād
ista-devatā
sāmprayogah.
from
svādhyāya
(arises) union
with one's
desired deity.

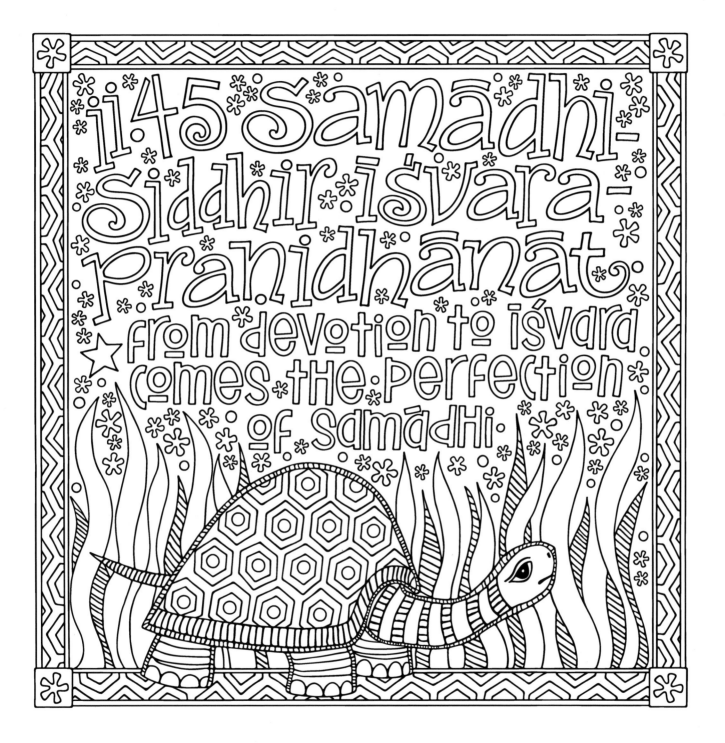

i.45 Samādhi-Siddhir·iśvara-Pranidhānāt

from devotion to iśvara comes the perfection of samādhi

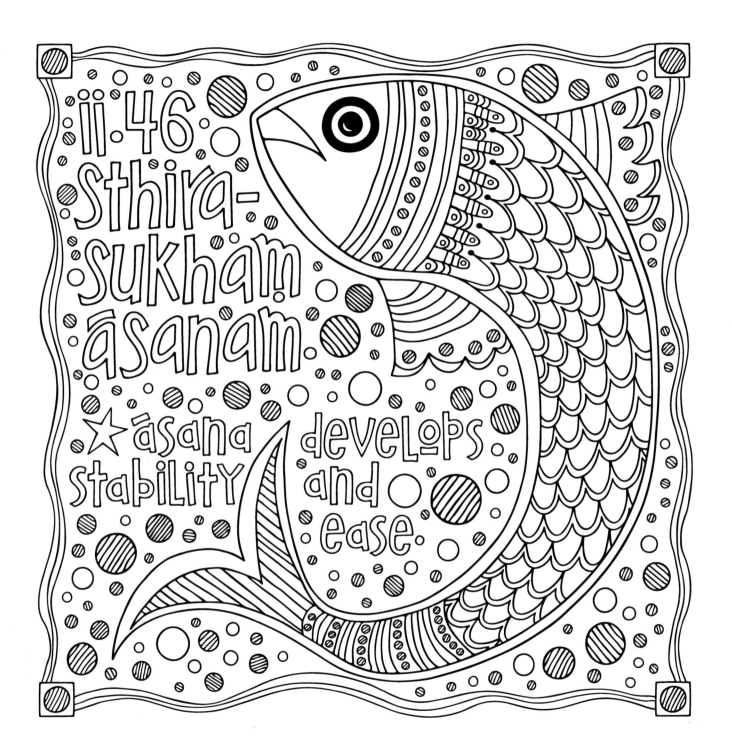

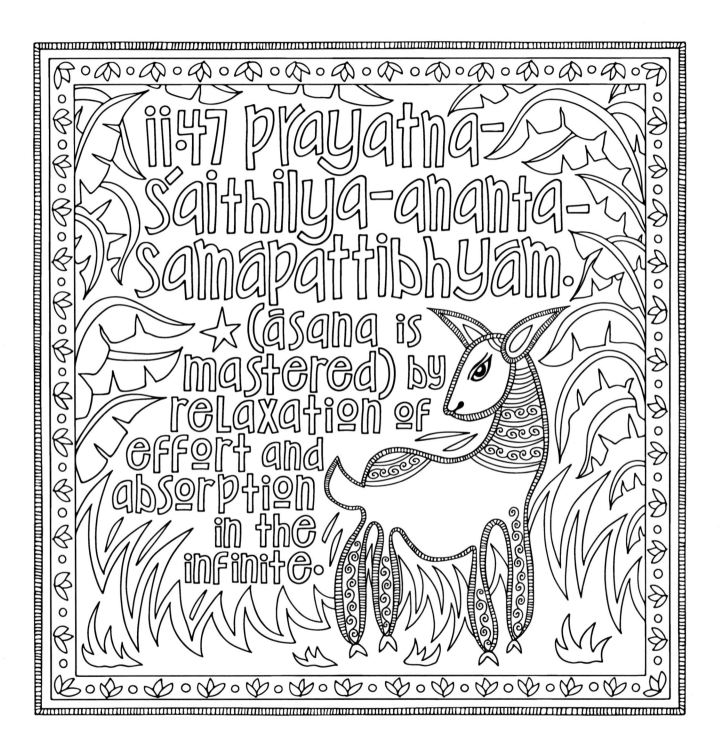

ii.47 prayatna-śaithilya-ananta-samāpattibhyām. ★ (āsana is mastered) by relaxation of effort and absorption in the infinite.

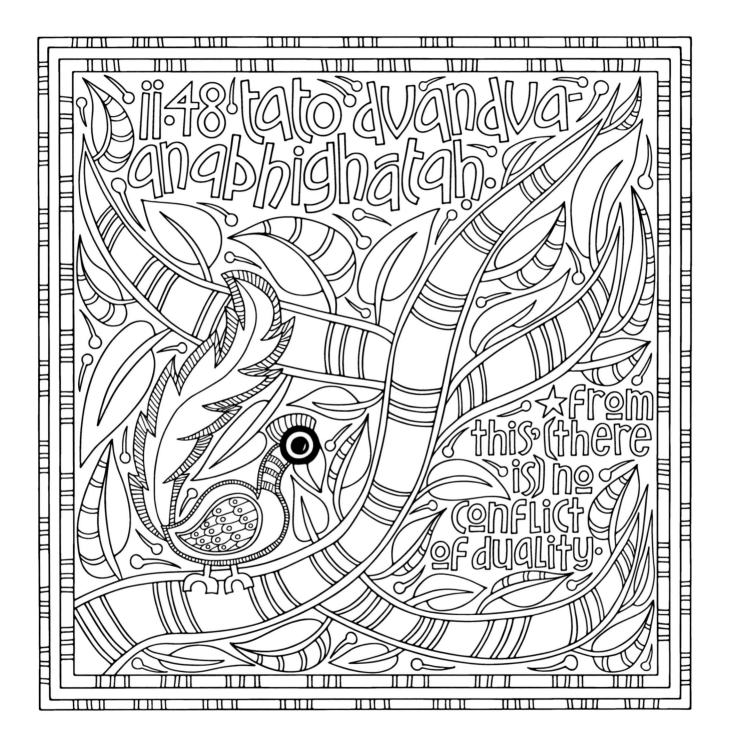

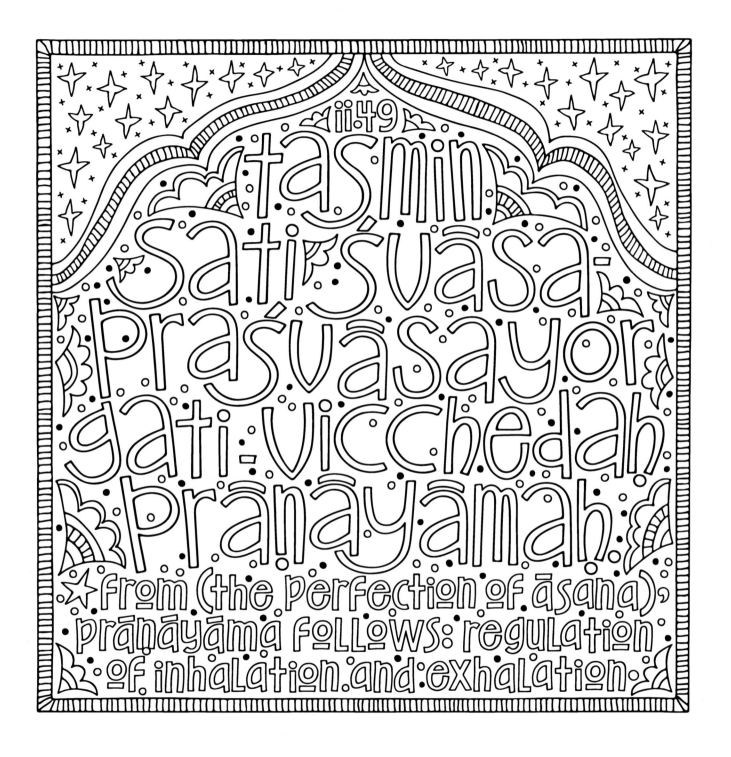

ii.49

tasmin
sati śvāsa-
praśvāsayor
gati-vicchedaḥ
prāṇāyāmaḥ

from (the perfection of āsana),
prāṇāyāma follows: regulation
of inhalation and exhalation

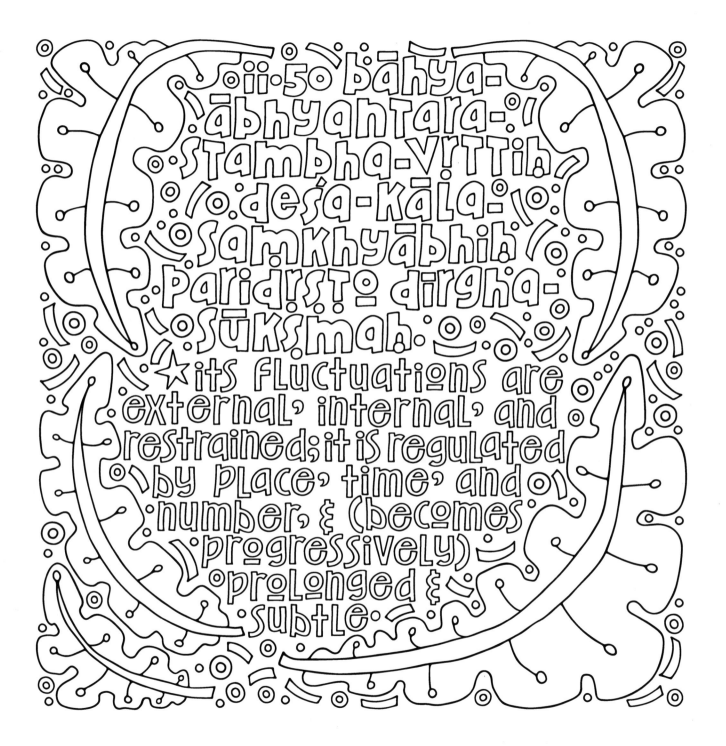

ii.50 bāhya-ābhyantara-stambha-vṛttiḥ deśa-kāla-saṁkhyābhiḥ paridṛṣṭo dīrgha-sūkṣmaḥ

its fluctuations are external, internal, and restrained; it is regulated by place, time, and number, & (becomes progressively) prolonged & subtle

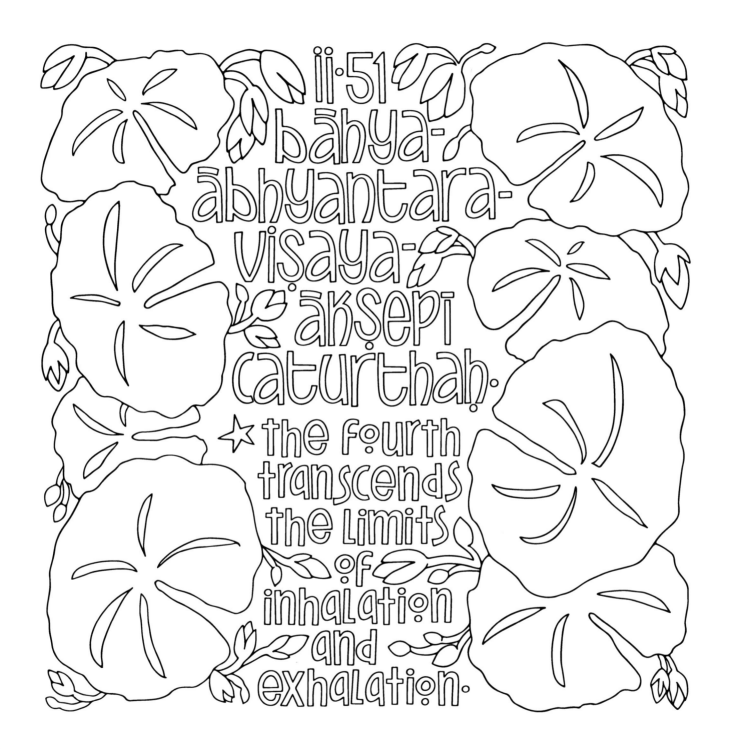

ii·51
bāhya-
ābhyantara-
viṣaya-
ākṣepī
caturthaḥ.

☆ the fourth
transcends
the limits
of
inhalation
and
exhalation.

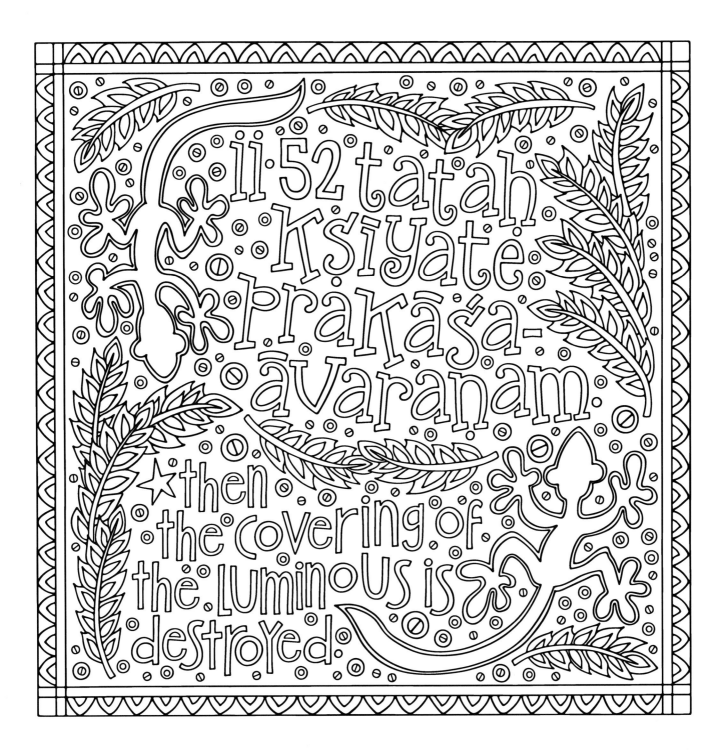

ii.52 tataḥ kṣiyate prakāśa-āvaraṇam

then the covering of the luminous is destroyed.

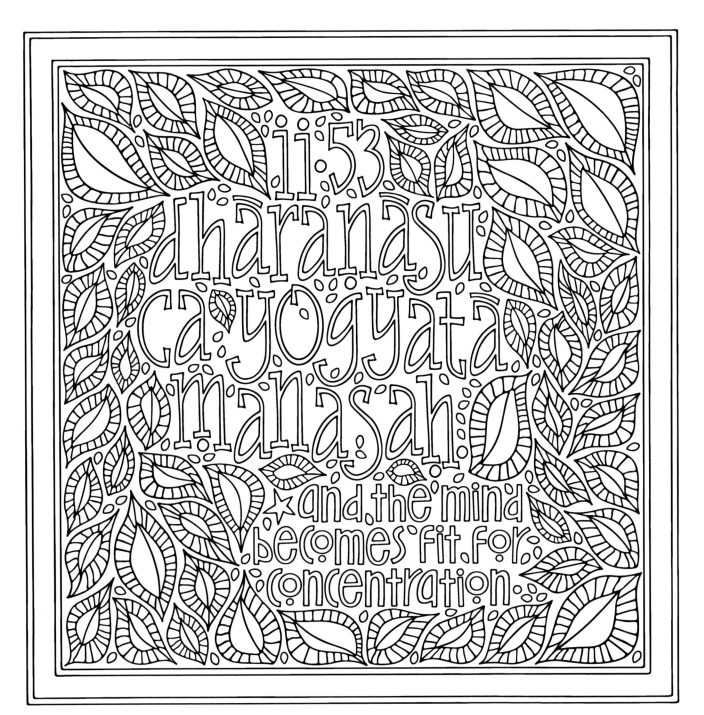

ii.53

dharanasu
ca yogyata
manasah

and the mind
becomes fit for
concentration

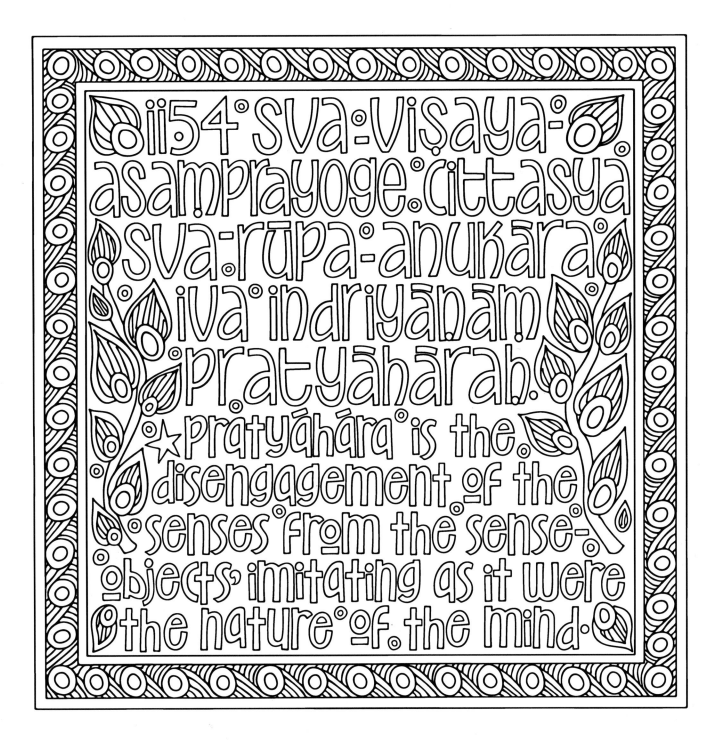

ii54 sva-viṣaya-
asaṃprayoge cittasya
sva-rūpa-anukāra
iva indriyāṇām
pratyāhāraḥ.
★ pratyāhāra is the
disengagement of the
senses from the sense-
objects imitating as it were
the nature of the mind.

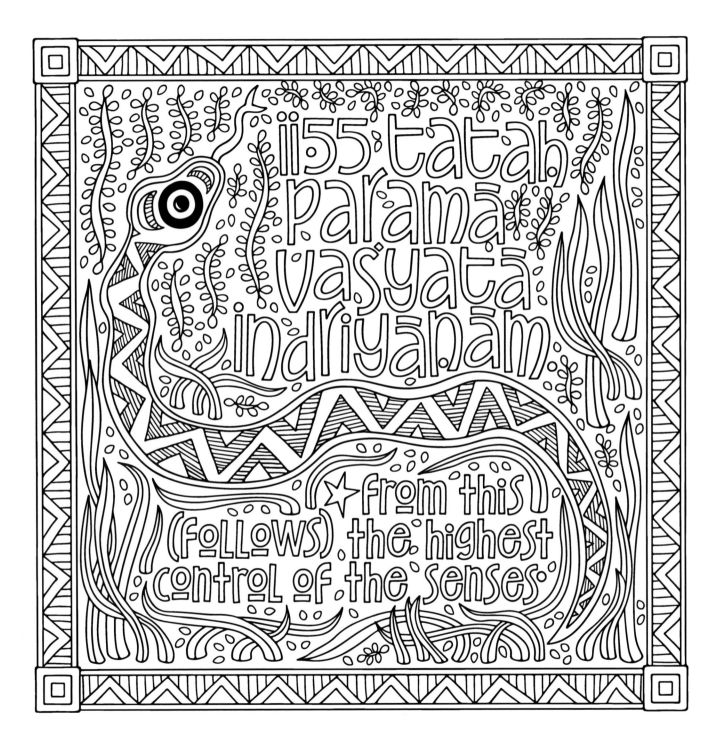

bibliography

Aranya, Swami Hariharananda, and P. N. Mukherji, et al. *Yoga Philosophy of Patanjali: Containing His Yoga Aphorisms with Vyasa's Commentary in Sanskrit and a Translation with Annotations Including Many Suggestions for the Practice of Yoga.* New York: State University of New York Press, 1984.

> This is definitely a study guide. It is meant to be patiently absorbed, bit by bit. This book provides Vyasa's commentary in the original Sanskrit and English, and deftly explains the *Sūtras* with a focus on the Samkhya philosophy that undergirds them. Not for the faint of heart.

Bryant, Edwin; Patañjali. *The Yoga Sūtras of Patañjali: A New Edition, Translation, and Commentary with Insights from the Traditional Commentators.* New York: North Point Press, 2009.

> This is another dense study. But unlike Aranya's *Sūtras*, Bryant's insights are more approachable. Bryant delivers a damn good scholarly treatise with a modern sensibility. The lengthy introduction on the history of yoga is invaluable.

Chapple, Christopher Key, and Yogi Anand Viraj. *The Yoga Sūtras of Patañjali: An Analysis of the Sanskrit with Accompanying English Translation.* Delhi, India: Sri Satguru Publications, 1990.

> A word-by-word analysis of the *Yoga Sūtras* with the Sanskrit word, its meaning, the source root, and grammatical classification. If you are a bit of a Sanskrit geek, or a lay etymologist, you will love this aspect.

Iyengar, B. K. S. *Light on the Yoga Sūtras of Patañjali.* United Kingdom: HarperCollins UK, 2002.

> There is no question that BKS Iyengar is one of the most important teachers of the yoga tradition. In this book, Iyengar does what he does best—distill the *Sūtras* down into a clear, practical, and applicable approach to modern life.

Prabhavananda, Swami, and Christopher Isherwood, et al. *How to Know God: The Yoga Aphorisms of Patañjali*. Vedanta Press, 1950/1983.

This is a great text for any beginner who is interested in learning more of yoga philosophy in order to deepen their spiritual practices. The beauty of this book is that it relates the insight of the *Sūtras* to other wisdom traditions of the world, making profound connections between Eastern and Western spiritual traditions. Like Swami Satchidananda's translation, it is delightful.

Ravikanth, B. *Yoga Sutras of Patanjali: Nature of the Mind, the Universe, and the True Self.* Berkley: SanskritWorks, 2012.

Ravi and I both studied with the same Sanskrit teacher, Dr. Ram Karan Sharma, and I can say with confidence that this translation is a hidden gem! It is easy to follow with illustrations that help to clarify the most complex philosophical points.

Satchidananda, Sri Swami. *The Yoga Sutras of Patanjali.* Yogaville, Virginia: Integral Yoga Publications, 1978.

There is a certain sweetness to the books translated by Satchidananda, and his *Sūtras* are no exception. His approach to the text is down-to-earth, reminding us that yoga is an every day, every moment practice. Sanskrit has a resonance all its own, and I appreciate that Swami Satchidananda presents the aphorisms in Sanskrit first with an English transliteration, and then his commentary. This is a very accessible text.

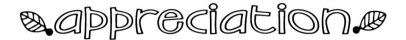appreciation

I have been so blessed to have had so many wonderful teachers in my life, and as I have said before, three titans stand apart from the many—Om Prakash Tiwari, a luminary in the promulgation of yoga; the late Dr. Ram Karan Sharma, a heavyweight in the world of Sanskrit; and the late Dr. Hilary Anderson, a champion of East-West understanding. I am forever indebted to this trinity of generosity and knowledge.

The design direction for this whole coloring book series and Blū Lotus would not have been possible without the guidance of Jenny Dupont. This is not an overstatement. Jenny helped me realize my design vision for this entire project, all the while creating a gorgeous website for Blū Lotus Publications. Plus, she's got a quirky sense of humor that I found necessary when working so closely together on my passion project. A huge thanks also goes to Tricia Counce, for her stunning color design of this book and her continuous enthusiasm for my endless stream of ideas.

A generous sense of gratitude goes to Timothy Tunnel and Sylvia Do Pico, whose insightful feedback and sage advice have been indispensable to me. Gratitude also goes to Karin Bauer and Mary Lou Song of Aspentri for helping me clarify my vision around Blū Lotus Publications. Their input was invaluable. A special thanks goes to Lloyd Rath, for his trusted wisecracks and his unflagging support; and to Blake Hallanan for her thoughtful feedback on this project.

My mother has always been my champion. When I was a child, growing up brown-eyed in a family full of blue-eyed folks, my mother would buy me brown-eyed dolls to make me feel special. When I was a young adolescent, she declared, "Nothing you do will ever surprise me." Not something you should ever tell a teenager, but in her way, she was acknowledging my particular zest for life. Needless to say, my mother has been an enthusiastic supporter of Blū Lotus Publications and this coloring book series of the Yoga Sūtras. I have dedicated this volume to her.

about the author

Like many people in the United States, Rebecca Polack's first introduction to yoga was at a gym—the YWCA in downtown Minneapolis. Yoga was still a foreign practice to most people 35 years ago, and yoga classes at the Y whetted Rebecca's appetite for a more comprehensive understanding of the practices. With that in mind, she quickly moved to study Iyengar yoga with William Prottengeier in 1987. After moving to New York City in 1996, she sought to deepen her practice of postures and breathing techniques at the New York Iyengar Institute with Genny Kapuler, the late Mary Dunn, and Judy Freedman.

Yoga was fast becoming a way of life for Rebecca, and New York City offered an exciting array of yoga schools. Eager to learn still more about yoga and its practices, Rebecca studied in depth with Cyndi Lee and Dharma Mittra. In 1997, she became a certified Yoga teacher through OM Yoga Center in accordance with the national requirements of Yoga Alliance. She studied Ashtanga yoga with Eddie Stern and Sri K. Pattabhi Jois, and took advanced teacher trainings with Rodney Yee, David Swenson, and Erich Schiffman. Rebecca furthered her studies with certifications in Prana Yoga with Dr. Jeffrey Migdow, MD, and Yoga for the Heart with Nischala Joy Devi, a yoga system based upon Dr. Dean Ornish's Program for Reversing Heart Disease.

The teacher appears when the student is ready, and that happened for Rebecca in 1997 when she met Om Prakash Tiwari, the highly-respected master of pranayama and Director of the Kaivalyadhama Yoga Research Institute in Lonavala. Possessing a wealth of knowledge about yoga, both culturally and historically, O.P. Tiwari imparted (and continues to impart) to Rebecca the nuances of the yoga practices and its philosophy. His teacher, the eminent yogi and freedom fighter, Swami Kuvalayananda, established the Kaivalyadhama Institute in 1924—the first institute of its kind in India and the world—to study yoga from a modern scientific perspective.

Since 1997, Rebecca has taught yoga in New York City and the tri-state region,

Minneapolis, Costa Rica, India, and now San Francisco. These days, Rebecca teaches small classes and one-on-one sessions with students looking to strengthen their practice in private—often working with beginners; people recovering from injuries; and those with special needs. She has also been involved in the teaching and training of new yoga teachers, with special emphasis on teaching pranayama. In order to create a "radically inclusive" yoga scene in NYC, Rebecca co-founded the New York Yoga Teachers Association in 1998 with Karen Safire and Cyndi Lee to promote conversation and community across the varied schools of yoga. She was the board chair for the first three years of the organization's operation.

In 2003, Rebecca moved to San Francisco to pursue graduate-level studies in yoga and South Asian philosophy. She holds a Doctorate in Philosophy and Religion at the California Institute of Integral Studies (2014) with a concentration in Yoga Studies. In addition to her academic studies, Rebecca has been blessed to study South Asian philosophy and Sanskrit in the traditional way—especially the *Yoga Sūtras* of Patañjali—with O.P. Tiwari, the late Dr. Ram Karan Sharma, and Shanta and Indira Bulkin of the Yoga Society of San Francisco. She has lectured on the modernization of yoga in New York City, Mumbai, Pune, Lonavala, and San Francisco.

Rebecca resides in San Francisco, and is currently is working on the third and fourth books of the *Yoga Sūtras* coloring book series, as well as a manuscript entitled "The Politics of Yoga: Swami Kuvalayananda and the Indian Independence Movement."